About the Author

Rob Kemp is a freelance journalist, and author of several books including *The Expectant Dad's Survival Guide*, and *The New Dad's Survival Guide: What to Expect In The First Year and Beyond*. He has written articles on the subject of pregnancy and fatherhood for a number of national titles including the *Guardian*, the *Telegraph*, *Men's Health*, *FQ*, *Pregnancy & Birth* and *Mother & Baby*.

THE
EXPECTANT DAD'S
SURVIVAL GUIDE

Everything You Need To Know

Rob Kemp

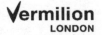
Vermilion
LONDON

Vermilion, an imprint of Ebury Publishing,
20 Vauxhall Bridge Road,
London SW1V 2SA

Vermilion is part of the Penguin Random House group of companies whose
addresses can be found at global.penguinrandomhouse.com

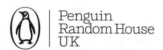

Copyright © Rob Kemp 2010

Rob Kemp has asserted his right to be identified as the author of this Work in
accordance with the Copyright, Designs and Patents Act 1988

First published in the United Kingdom by Vermilion in 2010

www.penguin.co.uk

A CIP catalogue record for this book is available from the British Library

ISBN 9780091929794

Printed and bound in Great Britain by Clays Ltd, Elcograf S.p.A.

Penguin Random House is committed to a sustainable future for our business, our
readers and our planet. This book is made from Forest Stewardship Council®
certified paper.

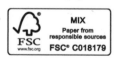

For every man who has heard those two magic words: 'I'm pregnant' . . . and immediately thought of two of his own.

Contents

In the Beginning

Dads aren't what they used to be. Within the space of barely a generation the role of the modern father and the duties and attitudes expected of him have changed beyond all recognition.

If you're able to, ask your own dad about his role in your birth. Ask him if he was at the birth, as in physically alongside your mother when your head popped out. Find out if he sat through birth-preparation classes during the pregnancy or if he recalls how he felt on discovering he was going to be a dad. You'll most likely discover that he certainly didn't cut the umbilical cord that connected you to your mum. He almost definitely never took a turn in feeding expressed milk to his infant son and he wouldn't have been seen dead strapping his newborn nipper to his chest in a fashionable, yet functional, papoose before heading off for a coffee morning during his paternity leave.

It's not because your dad was some kind of macho DI Gene Hunt character – though he may have dressed that way back then. It's simply because expectant fathers weren't expected to do such things.

But times have changed. If you're reading this I'm guessing that you're about to become a father for the first time and all of the above – and a whole lot more – will be expected of you. You're probably still trying to get your head around the idea. You're no doubt saying to yourself – and any mates who'll listen – that you're not ready for it. You're definitely wondering how it will affect you and what part you're meant to play in it all.

I know because I felt that way – and many of the new dads I've spoken to through my work with *Fathers' Quarterly* magazine did too. I didn't have a clue what I was meant to do. Half the time I didn't understand why my wife was acting the way she was. I certainly struggled to feel any bond or empathy with the thing growing inside her. I didn't even know if I wanted to be a dad. Even now, a few years down the line, I still have the odd day when I wonder if I'm really cut out for it all.

What I felt I needed at the time – and I've failed to see appear since – is some practical advice for the dad-to-be. I wanted something I could refer to in those dark, sleep-disturbed hours for some expert advice. I wanted to play my part – but I wasn't sure how to. In this book you'll find expert tips, in the main from a male midwife and father, Melvyn Dunstall, but also from obstetricians, psychologists and health-and-fitness specialists, plus a man who knows an awful lot about car seats.

The lifelong journey that is fatherhood begins well before your child takes his or her first gulp of air outside the womb. In a world where men and women share the benefits and burdens of being joint breadwinners the role of the modern dad has had to adapt.

We're now meant to 'be there'. We're expected to be supportive through the next nine months, to help with vital, life-changing decisions, to grow from lad to dad, to form a bond with our unborn baby and even have an opinion on such issues as disposable nappies or natural versus drug-assisted birth.

It's daunting, for sure, but it's not difficult to get up to speed on what's happening, what all the jargon means and what you should be doing. This book is designed so you can dip into it at any point during the pregnancy and early stages of your child's life and discover all you need to know to play your role.

And it's essential that you do, too. Research into the relationship between dads and their unborn babies shows that the earlier men get used to the role of responsibility, the sooner we act like dads, the more chance there is that we'll not only take to it but that we'll hang around long enough to see the job through.

The same research also shows that dads-to-be who are armed with the facts and involved in the process from day one are a lot less likely to suffer from depression later in life and a lot more likely to develop a strong connection with the baby.

Such evidence has led to a push, if that's the right term, among midwives and groups such as the National Childbirth Trust (a very useful charity providing expectant parents with advice, support and access to a shedload of quality second-hand baby gear) to get fathers more involved in the pregnancy process and early childcare. Don't be surprised if the midwife appointed to look after your partner – and the whole troop of health professionals that are about to enter your life – seem enthusiastic for you to do your bit. Hopefully this book will ensure that when you reply to their instructions with the line 'Yeah, I know that,' you won't be bluffing.

So, first off, congratulations. You've purchased, loaned, borrowed, browsed, thumbed through or been forced to read this book for one reason and one reason alone. You are about to become a father for the first time. You've heard the line 'I'm pregnant.' You're pretty damn sure it's your fault and you're now taking a peek at this in a section of the bookshop you've never been in before.

Consider this book your first as a new father. Each chapter roughly follows the pregnancy as it should progress. It'll give you an idea of how your child is developing in the womb, how your partner is feeling and why she's in the mood she is – and most importantly it'll give you the expert-sourced advice and tips you need to make the right decisions and noises. There will also be plenty of first-person testimony from fathers going through the same emotions and dilemmas that you will.

1
Discovering You're About to Become a Dad

Pregnancy: Weeks 0-8

While you and your partner contend with the initial shock of becoming pregnant, here's what the kid's up to. At this point the embryo inside her is growing. It will be about a quarter of an inch (5mm) in length by the sixth week – around the size of a Subbuteo footballer, but without the base! At this point the little life's basic nervous system is beginning to develop. The heart, brain and spinal cord are forming from around the fifth week onwards. Tiny buds that will become eyes, ears and limbs appear by the end of the eighth week.

HOW DO YOU KNOW YOU'RE GOING TO BECOME A FATHER?

Your partner may suspect she's pregnant. You too may have spotted some of the telltale signs in her. To indulge your detective fantasy a little further, look for clues such as:

The missed period

Admittedly it's not a clue that you'll easily discover off your own bat, but your ears should prick up if you hear her use this term on the phone or in polite conversation. It means that the womb lining that usually appears as her period once a month suddenly hasn't.

This may be because the egg that her body produces each month – and which your sperm may have now fertilised – is starting to become a baby. Once this happens it releases hormones that bulk up her womb lining and so stop it from leaking out each month as her period. Beware though, suspicious sleuth. According to experts such as male midwife Melvyn Dunstall some women can still have a very light period when they're pregnant. Others can miss a period but not be pregnant. Prepare for such false dawns happening a lot during pregnancy.

Her strange tastes

That's right, many women suddenly go off their favourite tastes. Tea, coffee, Pinot Grigio, cigarettes – it's a common indicator that things are stirring down below. Others claim to notice a 'metallic' taste in their mouth. If she hasn't just had a dental filling or left the teaspoon in the cup then Mothercare most likely awaits, mate.

Morning sickness

Now the clues are getting easier . . . A bit of a misnomer, this one, in that the spontaneous need to throw up can actually kick in at any time of day or night for her. Yet 50 per cent of pregnant women don't experience morning sickness at all. Be prepared for many of the preconceptions you have about pregnancy like this to be dashed. Those who do suffer some form of sickness usually do so during the first and second trimesters (the three-month stages of pregnancy).

As a father-to-be it's useful to know that stress can make her overly sensitive digestive system even more spontaneous – so anything you can do to keep her calm will combat morning sickness.

Be prepared to change your own eating habits, for a few months at least – and don't be surprised if she's also reluctant to cook, as even your favourite dishes suddenly turn into pungent triggers for her to spew.

The cravings

On the other hand, you could be lucky and find an early symptom of her expecting is a food craving for, well, chicken tikka maybe. As many as 90 per cent of expectant women experience a craving of some description – mainly in the first trimester. Some desire comfort foods such as mashed potatoes, cereals and bread. Such stodgy foods contain plenty of energy-giving carbs. Others crave stuff that isn't even food, including coal and clay. You may find yourself called upon to make a late-night dash to the supermarket, though your more helpful role will be in distracting her if the cravings she has are for stuff she really shouldn't be having. Take her out for a walk if your pregnant partner suddenly finds herself with a voracious desire for a Marlboro Light.

Total lethargy

An overwhelming fatigue during the day, which isn't helped by a need to pass water more often in the night. This tiredness will compound her mood swings, spontaneous tearful outbursts and sheer anxiety about the health of the baby. It can strike at any time in the next nine months – and beyond.

The breast engorgement

Another new term for you to use in Scrabble – it means the veins in her breasts show up more, her breasts become larger and her nipples may darken or become more prominent. This could possibly be the symptom we're most likely to take note of. It's an odds-on bet that it's a symptom we spot before even she does. Before you start thinking Christmas has come early, engorgement can make her breasts quite tender too – you may be told you can look but don't touch.

Of course these 'clues' are far from conclusive. That is why thousands of couples shell out on a bit of modern technology that has become the best way of discovering if you're about to become a dad for the first time.

HOW DO WE KNOW FOR SURE?

Most pregnancies are self-diagnosed at home using a test that detects a hormone called human Chorionic Gonadotrophin (hCG) in a woman's urine. The home pregnancy test kit is a mini-chemistry set that means women can confirm their suspicions without having a medical examination. They are sold at supermarkets and pharmacies – or free at some community contraceptive clinics and GP surgeries.

These devices – which have also revolutionised soap-story plotlines, often being found in the bathroom cabinet of teenage schoolgirls or supposedly 'barren' female characters – first changed the way a couple discovered that parenthood could be on its way in the 1970s. They're still the most common method of confirmation, either way.

Appropriately enough for some of us expectant dads, the kit itself is a dipstick-like tool. On to this a little drop of lady wee must fall. For the most part you're surplus to requirements at this point – but if nothing else the home pregnancy test kit is a gadget and one that provides an almost instant result, which is something that's always of interest to any bloke. And the result it reveals will seriously influence the next 50 years of your life, so it pays to know a little about how it works.

Did you know?

Taking the Pee

The method of checking a woman's urine to discover if she is pregnant dates back hundreds of years. A 16th-century pamphlet tells of 'piss prophets' checking the colour and consistency of urine passed by women thought to be pregnant. Some 'quacks' even added wine to it and observed the reaction the proteins in the pee had to the alcohol.

How does a pregnancy test work?

This hCG hormone is produced by tissue surrounding the embryo that eventually develops into the placenta. According to Melvyn Dunstall that hormone is detectable in a woman's urine usually from the day her period was due. As the urine seeps up the dipstick it passes through a layer containing antibodies that specifically bind to hCG, giving a positive reaction if hCG is present.

The most commonly available brands include Clearblue Pregnancy Test Kit, SureSign and the Twin pack pregnancy testing kit. (Twin in this case denotes two tests, not two babies on the way.) Once she has waved the stick into the mid-stream of her pee she has to wait a few minutes before checking the result window. In the case of the Clearblue kit she will most likely see a blue '+' or POSITIVE word in the result window. A '–' (minus symbol) will tell her she's not pregnant.

How accurate is it?

They're all at least 97 per cent accurate. So say the midwives. Some are so sensitive they can detect the hormone changes before the day her period is due – but doing the tests early runs the risk of 'false negatives'. (A false negative is – think about it – a positive.) A positive pregnancy test is highly unlikely to be wrong – but 'negative' results can be wrong. Aside from the major shock of later discovering that she is pregnant when she thought she wasn't, this can also lead to confusion about birth and conception dates. It'll add to those soap-opera cliffhangers too.

To get around this many kits come with two tests – allowing her to get a second opinion, as it were, within a day or so of the first. Ask any dads you know where they were when they found out they were about to become a father for the first time. If they weren't at work speaking on the phone to their partner, or at home on the sofa with a stiff drink in hand – then the chances are they were fairly close to a toilet door, on the other side of which was an anxious woman with her 'chemistry set' in hand.

This discovery may take place just as dawn breaks, since women who suspect they're pregnant are often advised to take the test with their first wee of the day. The thinking behind this is that urine is more concentrated at this point – and so will have a higher dosage of that telltale hCG in it. However, the time of the test is not that important since hCG will be present in urine regardless.

Did you know?

Rats! I'm Pregnant!

Scientists first carried out tests to identify the presence of hCG in urine in 1927. To test for pregnancy back then a woman's wee was injected into immature rats. If the woman was not pregnant, there would be no reaction. If she was, the rat would come into season, which it was too young to do naturally.

WHAT'S SO 'POSITIVE' ABOUT HER BEING PREGNANT?

Hearing the news that you're about to become a dad is something that will spark a different reaction from one man to the next. Those words 'I'm pregnant' will almost certainly throw up some feelings of anxiety. Your partner will have been weighing up the side effects it'll have on her life too before telling you – so don't be surprised if she's not able to provide all the answers to your questions there and then.

Don't worry if you're not turning cartwheels the moment you hear you're about to become a dad. Your response won't necessarily set a trend for the rest of the pregnancy nor the rest of your life as a father. Many men baulk at the idea initially. Several expectant fathers I interviewed attending an antenatal group conceded to me that they met the news with a mixture of elation ('I've done it!') tinged with an underlying – though rarely voiced – sense of impending doom.

There's bound to be some soul-searching on the part of both you and her – and you're not alone if you experience a sense of anxiety. According to psychologist Russell Hurn, who specialises in dealing with young fathers, this is often because stable, happy relationships are one thing – and babies are something very, very different.

Babies mean change – and we're not just talking about nappies here. There are some fathers who think their lives will carry on the same – according to Hurn these are usually the ones who get the biggest shock and have to adjust the most.

One common reaction among men is to – silently in most cases – question their own commitment to their relationship with the mother. Babies mean a level of responsibility that falls beyond a stable relationship, insists Hurn.

Questioning yourself and your ability to cope with the role of fatherhood is something that will happen to almost all of us – not just at this point but at varying stages through a journey that'll last a good few years. The doubts you have at this point can be aired – a trouble shared and all that – though telling your partner all about how you don't think you're 'up for it' isn't advisable. Sure, tell her you're anxious about the unknown, but to trade your deeper concerns or simply get some insight from other fathers who've been in your position try talking to:

- Your GP
- Mates, particularly fellow dads
- Men-only antenatal groups
- Online fatherhood forums

EXPECTANT DADS' EXPERIENCES

Discovery and reaction

A group of expectant fathers who attended an antenatal group in Richmond, Surrey allowed me to follow their progress from the early stages of pregnancy right through to the birth and beyond. Their insights will appear throughout this book.

'I can remember where I was, and what was said, very clearly. Sarah had missed her period, and took a pregnancy test. I was watching TV and was quite annoyed to be interrupted to be told that the test was positive. I don't think I really believed it was possible – I assumed it was a mistake. I didn't believe it was real until we had the scan.'

Dominic N

'I came home from work and she said, "We're a little bit pregnant." We'd not been trying and had both agreed to wait a couple of years, but I was pleased as well as scared. It felt

quite early but we are happy in our marriage, our home and jobs, so no reason to wait.'   Charley G

'Mel's monthly cycle runs like clockwork, so she knows when she is going to come on and usually does within a few hours of the same time the previous month. We had only been trying for a couple of weeks so when Mel came home with the pregnancy testing kit, I was a little sceptical. This was the evening of the day that she was due on and also the day before I had a work-related exam. I had worked pretty hard for the exam and was worried that the news (either way) would be very distracting. If it came up positive, I would obviously be ecstatic and if it came up negative I'd be a little gutted, even knowing that conception in the first month is pretty rare. I managed to convince Mel that we should wait until the following evening, just to be sure on her period and to allow me to concentrate on the blasted exam.'   Matthew D

'My wife did a pregnancy test and it was positive. We'd been trying for a long time, been to see a specialist, done all the tests. Everything was fine and her advice was "relax". We went to Paris on our anniversary, got drunk, had a great time . . . and a few weeks later she was pregnant. I felt like getting drunk again! I was overjoyed!'   Tom L

WHAT DOES MY REACTION SAY ABOUT MY ATTITUDE TO BECOMING A DAD?

'Is it mine?'

It's not necessarily an unfair or offensive reaction to the news – though your other half probably won't see it like this. A 2005 study by Liverpool John Moores University found that 1 in 25 fathers may not be the biological parent of the child they believe to be theirs. It's a statistic that's led to a rise in paternity tests after the birth of the baby.

The firm DNA Bioscience suggest up to 20,000 paternity tests are carried out in this country annually. But a 2014 review of studies and DNA tests, carried out by sociologists at Swinburne University in Australia, found that 'misattributed pregnancy' may only account for 1 in every 100 births.

'Are you sure we're having a baby?'

Also a fairly common response. And not unjustified since until your partner has taken a pregnancy test she can't give you a hand-on-heart guarantee. Even if she has, she'll only be 97–99 per cent sure. For many fellas 97 per cent isn't enough and, unless we have something in writing along with confirmation from a recognised health authority, a second opinion, a hearty handshake and pat on the back from congratulatory mates, a copy of the first scan and have witnessed our partner's changing shape and craving for marshmallows dipped in Branston first-hand, then we'll continue to question the existence of this so-called baby. By about the fourth month it'll have sunk in.

'How did it happen?'

OK, it's not such an uncommon reaction either and perhaps a recap of the events that led to you buying this book in the first place wouldn't go amiss.

Expectancy Explained

'Little Miracle' – How You Created Your Baby

If you're one of these 'how did it happen?' types then you should know that sperm are of course the starting point for us chaps in the reproductive process. Each month from your early teens onwards your testicles will club together to produce around 12 billion sperm in the area of your scrotum called the seminiferous tubules.

Over a 20-day period these immature sperm travel to an area at the top of your testes called the epididymis where they grow until called upon, as it were, to do their duty.

With your penis erect – and suitably stimulated – the green light is given to a batch of around 300 million sperm to travel upwards along a vein called the vas deferens tube, which connects your testes to a gland where it mixes with some fructose sugar and alkalines. The vas deferens, by the way, is the tube that is 'snipped' during a vasectomy, should you decide at some point that you want to stop using contraception but still enjoy sex without any repercussions.

The fructose sugar acts as a fuel. It sends your sperm into a 'hyper' mode, making them boisterous, energetic and likely to shoot off in any direction once let off the reins – you'll no doubt pick up where that link between sugar rush and kids first begins.

The alkalines act as a kind of deflector shield for your sperm. If you think that sounds pretty sci-fi then consider the fact that those alkalines are there to combat the acidic juices they come up against inside her vagina and uterus. And you thought it was just the *Alien* that carried that stuff around inside itself.

As the sperm, sugar and acid-busting super-juice continue their journey, they travel through your prostate gland. Here is added a milky substance that bonds it all together as semen. When you reach the point of climax you'll release those 300 million sperm plus the mix of fructose sugar, alkalines and 'semenal' solution – both well shaken and stirred – into her vagina. Or the 'brick wall' teat of a condom if this is just a trial run.

Described like this you're no doubt envisaging a 'geyser' of baby-making solution spewing forth from something akin to a runaway fireman's hose. But, according to scientists with one of life's less desirable jobs, the average man's measure of sperm on ejaculation adds up to between 1.5 and 5 millilitres. That's right, 20 days in the making, a diluting journey through your nether regions and an almighty cannoning from your penis at the end of a hard night's wining, dining, charming, persuading and possibly begging on your part – and all you've got to show for your efforts is a teaspoon's-worth of baby-making juice.

And yet it's still enough to conquer the challenges it faces once it's released into your partner. Your sperm have between 12 and 48 hours to find her egg and fertilise it. Simple, you may think, since despite the 'teaspoon' volumes, there are still 300 million of the blighters. But a whole host of obstacles – not least of all the acids – will be taking out your sperm left, right and centre from the start. Most of your semen will actually leak out of the vagina again within moments of landing there – not something you see highlighted on washing powder adverts, but a fact all the same. Only the strongest, healthiest sperm will head onwards up through the cervix into the womb and into the Fallopian tube.

Depending on the time of the month – if your partner is ovulating – she'll have an egg sat in that tube. When it's not fertilised the egg passes out of her vagina along with a temporary womb lining as part of her period. If there's an egg there around 200 sperm will be needed to dissolve the egg's protective layer and the best sperm will attach themselves to the surface of the egg. Then one single sperm will go on to fertilise that egg. And that's how the life you and your partner have created begins.

All of which brings us back to the fact box at the start of this chapter. By the fifth week of her pregnancy, when your partner may suspect that her missed period is a sign of something much, much bigger to come, that sperm-and-egg combination is an embryo – 5mm in length and triggering the production of hormones that create that 'Positive' sign on a home pregnancy test kit. The next step for her – and you – should you decide that this baby is for you will be the EDD.

WHEN WILL OUR BABY BE BORN?

The Estimated Date of Delivery (EDD) is the first in a long line of bouncing bundles of letters forming acronyms that you'll hear during your foray into fatherhood. Other shortened groups of technical terms you'll be mystified by include NCT (National Childbirth Trust), ICU (Intensive Care Unit), TENS (Transcutaneous Electrical Nerve Stimulation), MMR (Measles, Mumps and Rubella) and WTBHN (Wet The Baby's Head Night, a diary date you need to pencil in) – all of which will be covered later.

To discover the EDD your partner will have confirmation of the result of the dipstick self-test with a health professional.

She'll be given the choice to see either her GP or midwife. According to Melvyn Dunstall it's more commonly midwives, although there are a few GPs who like to undertake antenatal care – most women should be seen by the midwife at eight weeks and current NICE (National Institute of Clinical Excellence) guidelines recommend that the booking examination should be completed before the 12th week of pregnancy.

The booking examination is the first of around 10 antenatal appointments and scans that your partner will have if this is her first baby. She'll be asked about her medical history and her family's medical history (e.g. any abnormal births).

It's around this point that the current age of your baby – or more specifically its estimated due date (the EDD) – is delivered to you. This will be based on the calendar-tracking formula called Naegele's Rule – pub-quiz buffs take note. It was devised by Franz Karl Naegele, a German professor who published rules for midwives – including working out the EDD – in 1830 using a formula that's still in use today.

The rule estimates the EDD by adding a year to the first day of the woman's Last Menstrual Period (LMP) then subtracting three months and adding seven days to that date. This approximates to the average normal human pregnancy, which lasts 40 weeks (280 days) from the LMP, or 38 weeks (266 days) from the date of fertilisation . . . Confused? You're not alone. See if this helps:

```
LMP        = 8 May 2009
+1 year    = 8 May 2010
-3 months  = 8 February 2010
+7 days    = 15 February 2010 – that's when your baby is due
```

If all this looks too much like long division then get online to websites such as www.justparents.co.uk or www.emmasdiary.co.uk where a pregnancy-due-date calculator does all the working out, so long as you know the first day of her last period.

WHY IS THE EDD IMPORTANT TO ME?

It's tempting to answer this question with 'a big fat nothing' since it's estimated that, even after more precise ultrasound scans are used to work out the age of the foetus and delivery date, only 5 per cent of first babies actually arrive on their due day.

Around 15 per cent of children will be born premature (before the completion of the 37th week) – though first-time babies are more likely to arrive after the EDD. Knowing the EDD is useful for fathers-to-be since you can start thinking about the following:

Your paternity leave

Since this is the date your baby is expected to arrive you can roughly work out when you'll take your leave from work – handy if you've any long-term projects on the works wall-planner. You can also put one eye on when to get in your last holiday, long-haul flight, rollercoaster ride together – since from now on the milestone dates in her pregnancy are also ones where she can no longer do such things.

Attending scans and visits

With the EDD your partner's GP or midwife has a rough guide as to how old and what size the baby should be at differing stages of pregnancy. From this they'll be able to determine when your partner's due to attend scans and checks – it's therefore useful to you too if you're required to show willing and turn up with her. Though most women know their period better than they know their PIN, it'll only be when she goes along for the first ultrasound scan on her first antenatal hospital appointment that the pair of you will get an accurate idea of size, age and the date your baby is due.

Settling the debate

Any arguments regarding the conception and whether it's yours can be settled by the EDD. For example, how could it have been conceived around 11 April if you weren't released on parole until 2 June?

Expectancy Explained

Congratulations! It's a Blastocyst

During these first few weeks of its life the embryo will undergo a number of name changes. Of course, it won't know about them – they're obstetric terms used by the multitudes of medical people about to enter your world – and the likelihood is none of them would appeal to even the Gwyneth Paltrows of this world. These names include the *zygote* (OK, maybe that has a bit of a ring to it), which is the title for a single sperm that penetrates the mother's egg cell, and the equally catchy *blastocyst*. A *blastocyst* is when the *zygote* divides, creating an inner group of cells with an outer shell. The inner group of cells will become the *embryo* (third name), while the outer group of cells will become the membranes that nourish and protect it. By the most likely time of 'discovery' – eight weeks – the *embryo* will measure around 22mm (nearly an inch) in length from head to bottom. The face, feet and fingers begin to form and the internal organs are all developing (technically at this stage it's the foetus). By now the heartbeat can be detected on an ultrasound scan.

Fatherhood Starts Now

Pregnancy: Weeks 9–12

Looking at her stomach? Wondering what's happening in there? Well, from eight weeks onwards little nodules that become your nipper's fingers, thumbs and toes begin to grow. Bones begin to form and the ears start to develop too. Just four weeks later the foetus is fully formed – that means limbs, organs and bones are well developed and it'll be moving around, not that your partner will feel it yet, since despite all this it's still barely as big as your thumb in size at this point.

WELCOME TO THE WORLD OF 'TRIMESTERS'

Pregnancies are broken down into three 'trimesters' – basically three lots of twelvish-week blocks during which the medical experts expect mother and baby – and to a much lesser extent you – to be doing certain things. The first trimester covers weeks 0–12. The second is weeks 13–27 and the third is from 28 weeks up until birth – which in most cases occurs between weeks 37 and 41.

There's no marked difference between the end of one trimester and the start of the next and each woman's pregnancy is different with varying rates of growth and different reactions to symptoms. All you will notice as the dad-to-be when it comes to the trimesters is that medical advice means there are certain things that she can do in one trimester that she won't be able to in the next one. For example, long-haul flights aren't recommended in the first or the third trimester. In the first trimester there's a risk of miscarriage; in the last there's a risk that your child will be born in international air space.

Here though, roughly, is how the trimesters can best be used by fathers-to-be.

- The first trimester is a good time to start changing your habits – quitting smoking, getting used to the idea of fatherhood and preparing for the life change.
- The second is a good time for practical issues – such as sorting out your paternity leave and decorating the nursery (you'll discover your child's sex at the 20-week scan so can choose colour schemes at least).
- The third is the time to start rehearsing your role in the birth process and those first few weeks after the birth. It's the time when the antenatal classes kick in, when your partner will be giving up work and the pair of you will be panic-buying all the gear you need.

WHAT CAN I DO TO HELP HER IN THE FIRST TRIMESTER?

Following the revelation of that 'Positive' sign on the home test kit and you hearing the words 'I'm pregnant' there's a period of acclimatisation. You're both adjusting to the idea but you may only have each other to talk to about it if you're avoiding spreading the word until it's safe to do so.

For many expectant fathers this is Phoney War time. The 'Phoney War' is the name for the period in 1939 – after World

War Two had been declared – when the nation went into a bit of a panic. Anti-aircraft guns were set up, gas masks were doled out, sandbags were piled around shop entrances. But then nothing happened. No bombs. No gas. Nothing. The Phoney War didn't last long, of course – and nor will yours. Prepare for a bombardment of expenses, for missions to Mothercare, for scans, pregnancy books and magazines, strange people fondling your partner in the street and the endless conversations the pair of you only seem to have about 'the baby'.

For now enjoy the Phoney War and its silence and get into the mindset of being a protective, healthy new dad.

Essential chores make up the bulk of a dad's involvement in the first trimester. This may not conjure up images of kicking a ball around with your newborn son or enjoying that special moment when, for the very first time, your daughter points at a pigeon and shouts out 'duck' – but these chores play a part in the wellbeing of your partner and unborn baby. They include:

Clearing up after cats and dogs

You may shamefully recall at least one occasion when you pretended not to see what'd been left on the carpet in the hope that your girlfriend would take care of it – 'after all, it's her cat!' All that must change. The removal of any cat or dog crap that appears around your house or garden must be top of any daddy-to-be to-do lists. The reason is toxoplasmosis, a parasitic infection found in little Tiddles's deposits that can cause still-birth or miscarriage of human babies.

This is no reason to suddenly pack up the family pet and send it off into quarantine – but just do your bit to ensure your partner avoids coming into contact with its waste. If she does have to empty litter trays it's crucial that she uses disposable rubber gloves and that trays are soaked with boiling water for five minutes afterwards.

Doing the gardening

Pretty much the same reason as above. What cats can bury in the soil will do no end of harm to your unborn baby. Similarly, any plans you had to adopt an abandoned ewe or visit the local farm will need a rethink as sheep and lambs can also carry toxoplasma along with another miscarriage-inducing bug called chlamydia psittaci. Makes you wonder how they were ever allowed near Jesus's manger.

Handling raw meat

If you're a bit of a Jamie Oliver at home or a gourmet of the garden griddle during the barbecue season then you need to be aware that pregnant women can also catch toxoplasmosis from raw or undercooked meat. Around 350 cases are reported in England and Wales each year, but the actual number of infections could be as high as 350,000 with the majority due to undercooked or cured meat products.

Any symptoms of the disease in your partner would be fairly mild – such as a sore throat and a mild fever – but the real risk is posed to your unborn child, including miscarriage, or an increased chance of a child developing eye infections or having learning difficulties later in life. Prevention is crucial and you can play a part by making sure she and you wash your hands thoroughly after handling raw meat, and avoid cured meats, such as smoked ham.

Being vigilant when cooking

Meals may become a bit of a lottery as the hormonal hurricane going on inside her means that food she may have been desperate for when you started chopping it is met with a look of undisguised disgust when it comes to serving it up. It's just another example of how certain smells or tastes can spark bouts of nausea in the pregnant female. When cooking for her be especially careful to:

- Make sure that all meat is cooked thoroughly and is piping hot before eating it.
- Wash fruit, vegetables and salads before eating them.
- Be aware of danger dishes such as pâté and soft cheese such as Brie and Camembert. These carry a heightened risk of listeria infection, which can cause miscarriage.

Go easy with eggs

Appropriately enough since you've just fertilised hers, any that she eats need to be handled with care too. The risk of contracting salmonella food poisoning is higher in pregnant women because their immune system is not running at full strength. Though the salmonella bacteria can't harm the baby directly, health advisors recommend that pregnant women avoid risk dishes such as 'home-made' mayonnaise. Food Standards Agency advice for pregnant women is being reviewed after a 2016 report by the Advisory Committee on the Microbiological Safety of Food found that British eggs with the red lion mark carry such a low risk that vulnerable groups, such as expectant mothers, could eat them lightly cooked or raw in items such as mayonnaise. Check the FSA website for the latest advice or else be sure to:

- Boil a medium-sized egg for at least seven minutes.
- Fry eggs on both sides and poach eggs until the white is completely set and opaque and the yolk is firm: this will take about five minutes for a medium-sized egg.
- Store any eggs where they cannot come in contact with other foods, stick to the use-by dates and don't use eggs with damaged shells.

WHAT WILL SHE BE FEELING AT THIS POINT?

When it comes to pregnancy you may not be 'feeling it' yet, but rest assured she will be. During this first trimester some of the more common symptoms such as fatigue and nausea – for her, not you – can kick in quite severely. But because she may not show any outward signs of her pregnancy as yet, you may struggle to appreciate what's happening to her.

The first and final trimesters often prove to be the most problematic times for mothers-to-be – you'll find this rule applies to seemingly everything from flying to having sex, but the simple fact is, your child is growing inside her at a rapid rate. It'll indirectly eat what she eats, sap her energy and – at often unpredictable moments – will contribute to her feeling drained, irritable and subject to bouts of loathing towards herself, her 'bump' and you. A lot towards you as it happens.

She's going to get a lot more tired and anxious as time goes on, so it seems almost natural for the expectant dad to start playing a more active – supportive – role in the pregnancy at this point. If nothing else it'll get you out of that Phoney War mental state and get your mind focused on your role as a new dad.

It's almost as if Mother Nature wanted it to be so because it's at around this point that the good habits you create – and the bad ones you break – can be among the best things you do for the health of your unborn son or daughter. Setting up a routine of dad tasks now – playing a bigger part in keeping the house clean, for example – will make them all come a little easier when, eight months down the line, she's unable to do anything of any use to man or beast and you'll feel as if you're running the show single-handedly.

AM I FIT FOR FATHERHOOD?

It won't just be her doing all the huffing, puffing, carrying and pushing, no matter how much you think this pregnancy isn't going to change your life. You're going to be called upon to play your part in nest building, kid carrying and pram pushing for the next few years too. It's not necessarily a reason to hit the gym, if you don't already. In fact your existing gym membership may be one of the things you contemplate sacrificing in a bid to save money. Don't! Becoming a dad for the first time forces a lot of fathers into a timely assessment of their lifestyle and habits. Getting fit, working off any stress and tension on the heavy bag or simply having a place to escape to that isn't the pub are all good reasons for you to retain your workout routine or start one.

Should I quit drinking?

Only if you want to (highly unlikely; pregnancy usually has the opposite effect on the male of the species) or your GP advises it (not a common request, to be honest) or you think it'll help your partner too. If you're used to having a drink at home together don't be surprised if your determination to keep up the habit when she quits doesn't go down too well. Four reasons to think about your drinking now are:

- Antenatal experts maintain that making joint sacrifices – such as shunning old habits – is part of the bonding experience too.

- Show some empathy with your partner and reduce her feelings of nausea by cutting down on your drinking around her at least. Making up for it with the occasional blow-out on a Friday after work, however, is nothing to feel guilty about, since you'll find out soon enough that hangovers and new babies are a lethal combination.

- You could actually use this change of habit as a bit of a precursor for things to come. Finding new – booze-free – pastimes the pair of you can share will come in handy once your baby arrives. Also, count up how much cash you save from a week or two off the drink and look at the list of baby 'essentials' you're going to have to get in Chapter 6. This could be a good time to rein in that Peroni and whisky chaser habit you have.

- Get used to spending sober nights in because in the last month of the pregnancy you could be 'on call' for a hospital dash at any moment.

Should I quit smoking?

Doctors, midwives, pregnancy books, old wives, new mums and anyone with a vested interest or not will tell your partner that drinking and especially smoking during pregnancy is quite possibly the most directly harmful act a mother-to-be can do to her unborn baby. You can join this group in nagging your partner for sure, though you may find that through making changes yourself you'll help your partner change her habits.

How to wean yourselves off:

If you both smoke then you may be better equipped to quit than a smoker in a relationship with a non-smoker.

The START Way to Stop Smoking

There's a world of quit-smoking methods and techniques. This one forms part of some NHS cessation programmes.

- **S** = Set a quit date. Your partner and you will be getting increasingly familiar with calendars and dates right now so this shouldn't be a problem. Pick a land-mark point in the very near future and say that's it – no more after that.

- **T** = Tell family, mates and colleagues that you are quitting – any folk you usually cadge cigarettes off should be told. Maybe tie this in with your announcement to everyone about your impending new arrival.
- **A** = Anticipate and plan for the challenges you'll face while quitting. If you or she associate smoking with certain events or times of the day, e.g. at the pub, after dinner etc., look at ways you can break those routines and end that association with the fags.
- **R** = Remove cigarettes and other tobacco products from your home and car. Especially from your home. In fact stop smoking at home or around your partner even if you can't stop elsewhere.
- **T** = Talk to your doctor about getting help to quit. If you're going along to the antenatal checks with your partner use the opportunity to talk to your GP about a smoking cessation programme. They'll provide advice and quitting aids like patches or gum. You'll also get the lowdown on what the weed is doing to your seed – with the side effect fags can have on fertility it's a wonder any smokers become parents at all.

Why not just quit when the baby comes along?

It's understandable that you might want to cling on to the bad habits you hold so dear before you're forced to give them up for good. But the sooner you quit smoking the less risk there is of your unborn child suffering from its effects.

Exposing your baby to second-hand smoke increases the risk of low birth weight and Sudden Infant Death Syndrome (SIDS), more commonly known as cot death. Also, smoking around your partner makes it harder for her to quit.

Any moves you make will have a positive effect on your health and more importantly the life of your child. A recent study of 286 smoking fathers in the Midlands – interviewed when their infants were eight to 14 weeks old – found that 78 per cent had at least attempted not smoking at home – and 60 per cent reported successfully not smoking around their children. Among those dads in the study who did quit, key reasons for their success included not being heavy smokers in the first place and having a knowledge of what smoking can do to a child.

Knowledge such as this: research from the American Association for Cancer Research in Washington, USA found that 'the compounds associated with second-hand smoke can cause genetic damage and may be a prelude to childhood leukemia and other cancers'. This study found that pregnant women exposed to the second-hand smoke of family members (or friends or colleagues) pass some of the blood-borne chemicals to their unborn babies.

Not only that but other research – also from the USA, this time the University of Louisville – found that the levels of tobacco carcinogens, the cancer-causing chemicals contained in cigarettes, were four to five times higher in passive smokers' babies than in those of non-smokers. They were 10 to 20 times higher in the babies of cigarette smokers.

Did you know?

Smoke Gets in Their Eyes

Dutch research into tobacco smoke and exposure to children carried out by Reijneveld, Lanting and Crone found that excessive infant crying occurred more frequently among babies whose fathers (but not mothers, oddly) smoked 15 or more cigarettes a day.

SHOULD *SHE* STILL BE EXERCISING?

Becoming parents for the first time is no reason to suddenly cancel your joint gym membership or call a halt to those weekend runs or cycle rides. So long as she's not warned off it by her GP your partner should be able to exercise quite safely while she's pregnant. Most midwives will actively encourage her to stay active and exercise as much as possible as a means of dealing with the burden of pregnancy. However, she will need to get specific advice about exercise and may be warned off tougher regimens like marathon training if she has a low-lying placenta, high blood pressure or if she's having more than one child.

WHAT CAN WE DO TOGETHER TO ENSURE THE HEALTH OF OUR BABY?

The general medical advice is that moderate exercise – 30 minutes a day of working up a bit of a sweat – is generally thought to raise the chances of the pair of you having a healthy baby.

Use these moments as an opportunity to spend some time together and make plans. As the pregnancy progresses some pastimes – like your regular pub sessions – may have to go on the back burner as you look to save some money. Having a few healthy habits you and she can share could ease the pain of missing the pub.

Go swimming together

In the early months mums-to-be report finding swimming a fun way to keep in shape, but as the bump gets bigger and heavier then some women have difficulty with strokes such as the front crawl. Also, it's not quite the weightless experience you'd think it would be – some say it feels as if they're swimming downhill!

Still, the pair of you can get a bit of training in for that water birth if nothing else.

Join a yoga group

This'll tie in nicely with all those breathing exercises the pair of you do at the antenatal class when role-playing the act of going into labour. Yoga is said to help women deal with the discomfort of pregnancy – this is said mainly by people selling yoga courses, though some expectant women and midwives claim it boosts circulation and relaxation and relieves fluid retention. Your local yoga groups may even run classes you and your partner can attend with the birth in mind.

Keep on walking

Without doubt the cheapest and easiest exercise for the pair of you to do together right up until the birth is walking. Not hiking as such – you'll find that as time progresses your partner will find the act of strolling along the high street becomes a mammoth task – but walking together will help you both keep in shape. Just remember when you do to:

- **Take some water with you.** Especially when out in hot weather to compensate for the loss of body fluid during your walking exercise.

- **Know when to stop**. There's no need for her to push herself in the belief she'll be fitter for the birth – let her dictate the pace.

- **Take your phone.** Keep up the walking habit together throughout the pregnancy. But as your partner's due date nears it'll not only be tougher for her to walk very far, but there's also the risk that walking will bring on her labour. Have the maternity ward number stored in your phone just in case.

Get a 'man bag'

Or get used to carrying a bag of some description – ideally a rucksack or at least something you're comfortable with. As if Mother Nature once again planned it, the more pregnant your partner becomes the less she'll want to carry stuff when you're out together. As a result she'll jettison any excess baggage on to you. You'll need to help out carrying stuff after the birth, too – nappies, wipes, bottles (the burden of debt and responsibility). This job of becoming her sherpa during pregnancy prepares you in some way. Also, if you've got your own bag you'll feel less conspicuous than if you have to carry her pink floral number.

Did you know?

Did You Know? Fathers are Fitter

Fathers clock up an extra 352 hours more exercise in the years between their kid's birth and its 16th birthday when compared to childless men.

What exercises should I be doing?

According to one, progressive, fitness expert I spoke to pregnancy can be the perfect reason for a man to get fit. Jonathan Lewis, father of two and a physiotherapist and trainer with London-based Balance Physiotherapy, insists the combination of a new life stage and the growing physical demands the dad-to-be faces makes this an ideal time to get into shape.

Lewis has devised a few exercise moves with expectant dads in mind. These are exercises you can do at home when you have a few spare moments, designed to raise your heart rate and use your own body weight to work your muscles.

Key to the convenience of these too is that they're floor-based – the only piece of equipment you may want to use (or snaffle off the missus) is an exercise mat – especially if you're working on bare floorboards. Lewis's fitness-for-expectant-fathers drill begins with simply getting down on the floor and doing:

Pregnant man's press-ups:

More commonly known as the 'Hindu push-up'. Start in the press-up position but instead of doing the basic up-and-down motion you raise your backside in the air then 'swoop' down with your chest so it almost touches the mat, before returning to the start and performing another 'dive'.

The idea, according to Lewis, is to go as low as possible, taking the head, chest and then belly as close to the ground as your strength and mobility allow.

These moves will work a range of muscles around your 'core' – the stomach and lower back. As a new dad you're going to be doing a lot more lifting of car seats and buggies as well as bending to change nappies – the stronger your core is, the easier these chores will be. You'll also cut your risk of straining anything. Believe it or not, 'baby injuries' are not uncommon among new fathers called upon to perform lifts or stretches their bodies are not used to.

Some GPs actively encourage new parents – both mums and dads – to do Pilates or similar muscle-stretching moves in the build-up to the birth. It's because the furniture shifting and weight-bearing that pregnancy brings lead to an increase in proud first-time fathers and mothers complaining to their doctors about bad backs.

Delivery room deep squats:

Another simple but effective drill. It's a move that will replicate some of the movements you'll be making when your child is born – it's also an exercise that will improve your fitness and stamina levels for the upcoming months.

Adopt a squat position. Lewis suggests you open your stance to allow you to sit your hips backwards and sink as low as possible. As you squat up/down maintain a straight line between toes, ankles, knees and your open hips. Losing alignment causes weakness and leaves your joints vulnerable to strain and overuse. Try to keep your weight on the heels and drive strongly back up.

At the top of the squat movement immediately step your left leg back to the left – you should sink into your right hip, ensuring your knee doesn't push forward off your toes.

The right leg is in control, the left leg provides balance. Drive up through your right heel and then immediately step back with your right leg to the right. Squat, step left back (works right), step back right (works left), repeat.

Pre-natal papa plank:

Again an anytime, anywhere exercise which you only need a floor to perform.

Get down on all fours in a press-up position. Hold your body straight – with your stomach off the ground – supporting your torso with your elbows and toes. Now tense your abdominals – stomach muscles – and try to keep a straight neck, flat back and legs for a count of 10 to 15 or up to 30 seconds. Once more you're hitting that key 'core' area and you can progress to holding the plank position for longer time periods as you get more accustomed to it.

WHEN DO I TELL PEOPLE I'M ABOUT TO BECOME A DAD?

In the terms of the epic pregnancy journey you're only just out of the starting blocks. This is an uncertain time – around 25 per cent of pregnancies end in miscarriage during the first 12 weeks.

Many couples don't tell their friends and family until they have had their first (12-week) or even second (20-week) scan when they find out the sex of the baby too.

Breaking the news of your impending fatherhood can be tempting from the very first moment she reveals the news to you. But HOLD YOUR FIRE. Other reasons why it's imperative that you don't start texting the boys in the Sunday team the moment her test turns to positive are outlined below:

You've got to be united

Sit down together and draw up a list of who you're going to reveal your wonderful news to and when you're going to tell them. As keen as you may be to announce it to the world, think about maybe telling close relatives at first – if anyone. There may be people the pair of you should be sensitive about telling – previous partners or children from other relationships. Think about how you'd like to be told if it were your close friends, or family, or your own kids telling you. Face to face would be ideal . . . Facebook, not so good.

You need to get used to it

As soon as the news gets out among friends and family that you're about to become parents your lives begin to change. All talk turns to that of 'the baby'. Gifts start appearing and cluttering up the place. The question 'thought of any names?' takes on a sinister element when it's the likes of Uncle Rumbold or Aunt Maude asking – with one eye on you naming your kid after them. Ideally take some time to savour the news yourself. Celebrate in your own way and get used to the fact you've created this new life – before all hell breaks loose.

You may want to wait

Problems can occur. As the Baby Stats at the start of this chapter confirm, at this stage the life you've created is ultra-fragile, and if you've experienced a miscarriage before the risk is higher of it happening again. Many couples wait until 'safer' landmarks before letting on to others.

You need to know details

I myself couldn't wait to tell the world the news. My wife phoned me from the GP's surgery on the day her pregnancy was confirmed with the caveat 'Don't say anything to anyone yet though; it's bad luck to tell people this early.' By lunchtime I was in the pub around the corner from work accepting back-slaps and handshakes between congratulatory pints. When you do decide to tell the world, at least have something chewable to tell them. Both male mates and female friends will immediately ask: 'How far gone is she?' 'When's it due?' 'What do you want – what does she want?'

A tip: have these answers in place and do not follow my example.

WHEN SHOULD SHE TELL WORK?

Company policies regarding maternity and paternity leave will vary vastly, but your partner will – generally – need to notify her workplace of her impending motherhood 15 weeks before the due date in order to arrange her leave. She does not have to tell her employer any earlier than that but most mums-to-be do – not just because they'll probably have guessed as she wobbles around the office, but as a courtesy to the employer and in order to take time out for antenatal checks, to rearrange work patterns and to ensure she qualifies for Ordinary Maternity Leave (OML). OML is for 26 weeks while a further 26 weeks' Additional Maternity Leave (AML) is also currently available to many new mothers – one year in total.

How can I help her at this point?

A few factors to consider when she books her time off work (she'll probably ask your advice or want some support). Consider how YOU would feel about taking a year out of work. OK, once you've uncorked the champagne at the very idea and got over the dreams of backpacking through Borneo or following the Barmy Army around the West Indies, consider some of the genuine concerns experienced by women taking maternity leave.

How would you feel about losing ground or having someone else covering your year off – and possibly being seen to be doing a better job than you?

How would you feel about missing out on the daily gossip, gags and social networking that goes on around your firm?

How would you feel about not having the structure that comes with work – the day-to-day routine that you may curse but which has become a reassuring habit too?

Your partner's anxieties during pregnancy may well include her perceived loss of status – especially if she decides to quit work completely. She may be wondering how she'll fare spending her days after the birth with only a mini-version of *you* to communicate with. One that barely speaks and only wants her when it's feeding time or when it wants to go to bed. (OK, maybe that sounds too much like a mini-you, but you get the idea.) Work is such an integral part of our lives and who we are that giving it up – even if it is only temporary – is bound to make her anxious.

Expectancy Explained

What You Need to Know about Her Leave

After nine months at home with the baby around 65 per cent of the 400,000 UK women on maternity leave each year will go back to work. By the time the child is 18 months old that figure rises to 80 per cent. However one 2009 study, by the Economic and Social Research Council, found that one in four soon-to-be dads had the wrong idea about their partner's intentions after the baby is born. She may say she's definitely going back to work at some point – but be prepared for that not to be the case. According to the ESRC research most new dads supported the mother's decision – even if it wasn't what they expected. Childcare difficulties, new job structures after the birth and a simple change of heart were all listed as major reasons why around one in five mums decide not to go back to work.

She needs to let her employer know when the expected week of childbirth is (EDD) and when she wants her maternity leave to start.

She can choose when to start her maternity leave. This is usually a month before the baby is due, though it can be any date from the beginning of the 11th week before the week the baby is due. (By law she can change this date – as long as she gives her employer 28 days' notice.)

In terms of going back, she can change the date of her return to work, as long as she informs her employer eight weeks in advance.

If she decides not to return to work at the end of her maternity leave, she's entitled to continue to receive her full amount of statutory maternity leave and pay as long as she gives her employer at least the notice required by her contract or, where there is none, the statutory notice.

WHY DOES SHE HAVE TWO TYPES OF MATERNITY LEAVE?

There's Ordinary Maternity Leave (the first 26 weeks of her Statutory Maternity Leave) and Additional Maternity Leave (the last 26 weeks). Unless she's agreed it in advance, her employer will assume that she's taking all 52 weeks of her Statutory Maternity Leave.

If she wishes to return to work earlier than that – for example, when her Statutory Maternity Pay ends – she must give at least eight weeks' notice.

WHAT PAY IS SHE ENTITLED TO WHEN ON MATERNITY LEAVE?

Statutory Maternity Pay (SMP) is paid for up to 39 weeks. She should get:

- 90% of her average weekly earnings (before tax) for the first 6 weeks
- £139.58 or 90% of her average weekly earnings (whichever is lower) for the next 33 weeks

SMP is paid in the same way as her wages (eg monthly or weekly). Tax and National Insurance will be deducted.

If she takes Shared Parental Leave – this involves you too, we'll come to this soon – she'll get Statutory Shared Parental Pay (ShPP). ShPP is £139.58 a week or 90% of her average weekly earnings, whichever is lower.

EXPECTANT DADS' EXPERIENCES

First Few Weeks

'She has been great compared to some of the other stories I heard about. The biggest surprise was that she started drinking beer and liking soup – which she didn't before.'   Tom L

'The hardest part of the first trimester has been the feeling that I cannot do anything to help with her discomfort. Dealing with the moods was pretty tough too; I had to keep reminding myself that this was pregnancy-related and that she didn't really hate me! Thankfully that didn't last too long.'   Matthew D

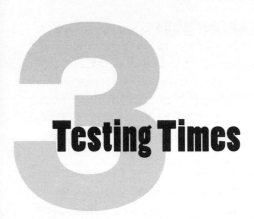

Testing Times

Pregnancy: Weeks 13–16

During this time the embryo will 'Supersize' by almost four times its current dimensions – even so it'll still measure only around 3½ inches (85mm) in length at the start of this month and around 5½ inches (140mm) by the end of it. It'll weigh around four ounces (100g). The baby's rapid heartbeat is now detectable through a device in the form of a tube or monitor with earphones attached called a doppler. In some women this three-month stage is when the first signs of 'the bump' appear. At 12 weeks your partner is already a third of the way through her pregnancy and at the end of the first 'trimester'.

WHAT DO I DO WHEN SHE HAS THE 'SCAN'?

The short answer to this is to do everything in your power to go along with her and be there too. For almost all new fathers the first time they actually see the CCTV-style 'proof' that they have created another life is a memorable moment, as we'll find out later from some expectant dads.

Your partner is required to attend an ultrasound scan at the hospital she's booked into or in some cases at a GP's surgery. Ultrasound scans have been in clinical use since 1960.

There are no known risks to them, though you and she may well feel a little anxious before going along – especially since the wording on the paperwork explains that these scans are designed to pick up on bad news as well as good. Even though you'll be given a still picture – a fuzzy, often indecipherable image of your baby in its very early stages – to take home with you, it's really nowhere near as good as catching it 'live'.

This 12-week scan is one of a number of tests and checks she'll go through during her pregnancy (there's a list of these below). This first scan is mainly used to check the EDD (estimated delivery date) and to see how many babies she's carrying in there, to check the growth and discover if there are any initial signs of physical abnormalities. The specialists know that this scan can reveal some serious defects. You now know this too. Most importantly, your partner knows this. Since worrying about her baby is something that she will do from now on and for the next forty-odd years at least, it'll be incredibly useful on your part to do the following:

Go along too

There are at least two routine scans that you'll need to attend and the first scan – when screenings for abnormalities or birth defects are carried out – is one of them. In most cases the news is good and it's a great opportunity to see your kid for yourself for the first time – then bore your workmates senseless with the scan pictures when you return to the office.

Ask for clarification

Take on the role of chief interrogator during any medical check-ups or scans you attend. Take note of any comment or observations the sonographer (person doing the scan) makes says and ask for clarification about anything you're not happy about and/ or don't understand at the end of the scan. Usually if a sonographer finds anything they're not sure about, or if you as parents have questions they cannot help with, then you'll be referred to see an obstetrician – the hospital specialist dealing with pregnancy.

Reassure her

Act as a calming, reasoned voice of comfort whenever she's getting worried about the checks or the results of the ones she's just had. You'll be anxious too, naturally enough, and it won't help either of you to bottle up any fears or concerns (just make sure you pick the right moment to express yours).

Expectancy Explained

What's Worrying Her?

At this stage a whole world of concerns will be filling her head including 'My bump is too small.' Remind her that it's not until you have a more detailed scan (at around 20 weeks) that you will know for sure how things are progressing. Also first-time mothers with taut stomach muscles don't show as much as the growing baby doesn't stretch the womb so much. Tell her that – she'll thank you for what could be the first complimentary thing you've said about her figure in years . . .

WHAT OTHER CHECKS WILL SHE HAVE?

Seemingly more than a rocket ship at take-off – in the vast majority of cases these are over in minutes and the news is good.

Confirmation of conception

According to Melvyn Dunstall modern ultrasound can detect a gestational sac (the beginning of a baby in layman's terms) within 18 days of fertilisation. Your partner will take a DIY test, then visit her GP, who may arrange an ultrasound.

Dad goes too? Not necessary.

Non-invasive prenatal blood test (NIPT)

Recently OK'd by the national screening service and still being rolled out within the NHS, this new test screens her blood for any trace of the extra chromosome 21, which causes Down's Syndrome. If the test is positive, doctors will suggest a further amniocentesis test.

Dad goes too? Not necessary.

Chorionic villus sampling (CVS)

A test designed to check for abnormal chromosomes or genetically inherited diseases such as cystic fibrosis or muscular dystrophy. Similar to an amniocentesis test – where fluid is extracted from the sac of fluid surrounding the foetus – it's performed at around nine to 11 weeks, and done only if your partner's GP feels she needs it.

Dad goes too? If you can, yes.

Twelve-week scan

Also called the nuchal translucency scan (by those in white coats), this is usually the first time parents actually see the baby. So the bonding can begin . . . and the rows over whom he or she looks like.

Dad goes too? Yes.

Alpha-fetoprotein test (AFP)

This blood test is usually done as part of a routine checkup and can help detect any risk of spina bifida (a rare, paralysing defect in the spinal cord) in your baby.

Dad goes too? Not necessary.

Amniocentesis (Also referred to as amniotic fluid test or AFT)

Carried out between 15 and 20 weeks on women with an increased risk of having a baby with Down's syndrome or spina bifida. It's not compulsory and some mums who are offered it refuse because there's a 1 per cent risk of a miscarriage occurring as a result of this test. Fluid is drawn from the sac surrounding the baby and sent away to be checked, so there is a wait for results.

Dad goes too? Not necessarily; it may be a lot more helpful to your partner to be around when she's getting the results.

Twenty-week scan (Also called mid-pregnancy scan)

This is the one where you can find out your baby's sex (we'll discuss the pros and cons of this in Chapter 5). If you want to know if you're having a boy or girl, ask. Officially the staff won't tell you unless you want them to. You can try guessing, but sonographers work pretty fast and it's not easy to tell a boy from a girl at that size anyway. Unusual abnormalities like a cleft lip can be detected at this scan.

Dad goes too? You betcha.

Urine and blood samples

A pregnant woman's pee reveals a myriad of medical insight. The presence of sugar in her urine could be a sign of pregnancy diabetes. It's a temporary condition usually controlled through a change in diet, though sometimes injections of insulin are required. Tests can also expose any risk of a side effect to pregnancy called hypertension. Blood tests will show her blood group – no surprise there – but are also designed to combat a possible clash of blood groups between mother and baby. Around 15 per cent of mothers are in the group rhesus *negative*. If she is but her baby is rhesus *positive* the mother's body may view the baby as an infection. To prevent this, all rhesus *negative* mums are now offered 'anti D' injections.

Dad goes too? To view a urine sample? Only if you're into that kind of thing . . .

Expectancy Explained

What is Pre-eclampsia?

Pre-eclampsia is an illness that affects women only during pregnancy – as many as 70,000 in the UK – which can often result in the placenta not working properly. This restricts the baby's food and oxygen supply and hinders its growth. The chances are it will have been diagnosed via blood and urine tests taken during your partner's antenatal visits and treated with drugs to lower her blood pressure. Other symptoms can include severe headaches, flashing lights or spots before the eyes, and stomach pains. It's estimated that around 1,000 babies die each year because of pre-eclampsia (NHS 2016).

Expectancy Explained

Antenatal Checks, Fathers and the Law

Scans really are an incredible, moving and often bonding experience for expectant dads to attend. Health experts, midwives and a whole lot of new and expectant dads will tell you that it's crucial for you to do all you can to make it to the scans at least. Talk to your workplace HR department if you're unsure of how to go about taking the time off to support your partner during her pregnancy. Pregnant women have a legal right to paid time off for antenatal care – which can include antenatal classes if they've been recommended by a doctor or midwife. As the father or pregnant woman's partner you have the right to unpaid time off work to go to two antenatal appointments. (So long as you are an employee or agency worker with 12 weeks' service doing the same kind of job with the same hirer.) After your child is born you have a right to request flexible work. For more information check out www.gov.uk/flexible-working.

In case you can't go to 'the big one' or you just want a heads up as to what it entails, here's the lowdown on the ultrasound.

WHAT HAPPENS DURING THE ULTRASOUND SCAN?

This could well be the first time you and your partner have attended a hospital together (except that trip to the STD clinic together a few years back, but we won't go into that right now), which could make this first scan an interesting experience in itself. It will prepare you – a little – for the dealings you're going to be having with health professionals over the next few months and after the birth.

On the whole the scan passes pretty quickly and almost all parents' experiences of dealing with doctors, midwives and obstetricians are great. The flowers, chocolates and thank-you cards dotted around the maternity ward will attest to this. But if you or your partner have any concerns then don't be afraid to speak up or ask for another opinion.

As the father you'll go along to this first scan to comfort her, to ask any questions that come to mind and above all else nod your head, say 'amazing' and where possible pretend to see the image that the sonographer tells you is your child. Don't worry too much about knowing what the sex of the baby is right now. If it's your partner's first (12-week) scan there's no way of telling if it's a boy or a girl anyway – the earliest a baby's sex can be determined is from around 16 weeks. Aside from that, sit back and enjoy the show as your partner:

- Lies on a hospital trolley/movable bed while a sonographer – usually female, though not always – smears a conductive clear jelly over her exposed stomach.

- Feels a bit of a twinge as the sonographer starts moving what looks like a karaoke mic on the end of a hose through the mulch of jelly on her belly.

- Looks mystified at the TV screen beside her while the sonographer explains how this contraption seemingly made up of U-boat-detecting sound waves being bounced around her abdomen is creating a picture of your child-to-be.

- Also looks anxious and squeezes your hand a little as the 'mic operator' performs a series of clicks taking measurements of your baby's head and limbs – when they finally manage to detect them it.

- Finally appears relieved when it's over – then pissed off that all she's given to remove the goo from her belly is a couple of sheets of harsh blue NHS standard sandpaper towels.

The whole thing will last around 20 minutes. The sonographer's reactions and utterances during the scan shouldn't be taken to mean that you have anything to worry about. They may simply be struggling to get a clear picture – remember, your baby at this point isn't much bigger than your middle finger – or else they're thinking about what they're going to have for lunch. Any problems relating to the scan or any questions you have should be discussed with your partner's GP or the midwife or obstetrician looking after you.

EXPECTANT DADS' EXPERIENCES

The First Scan . . .

Seeing the child you've created moving around for the very first time can be a rewarding and emotional experience – capable of bringing a tear to the eye of the most macho of men. As a result it's not necessarily something your mates in the pub may openly share – but thankfully a few expectant dads were willing to share the experience with me:

'The first scan was quite emotional. I had expected to see a blob on the screen and didn't expect to distinguish the baby clearly. In fact we could see the baby very clearly, particularly when he moved. This was probably an important thing for us to start getting used to having a baby, not a pregnancy. It was a big relief to find out that everything was OK and the baby was healthy.'

Charley G

'First scan was amazing, I didn't really know what to expect, I thought it was going to be a load of fuzz on the screen that we wouldn't be able to make head or tail of. As it turned out the first thing we saw was a little face looking out at us. I sat there, holding Mel's hand, with a perma-grin etched into my face and tears streaming down my cheeks from unblinking eyes. It was awesome!'

Matthew D

'The first scan was little more than a splodge on a screen, but it was amazing to see what was apparently a heartbeat but which looked more like a unicyclist.'

Dominic N

Can I get a picture from the scan?

You can. Some hospitals will give one to you for free. Others will charge a token fee of £1 per picture. If you ask for several shots you may be charged more than that. It'll make a wonderful keepsake and you'll be thrusting it under the noses of everyone you've told the news to at the first opportunity – but **ON NO ACCOUNT SHOULD YOU LAMINATE THE SCAN PICTURE.** The pics are produced on heat-sensitive paper and laminating it will simply destroy the image. Instead photocopy it or scan it and make copies if you want them.

Should we go for 4D?

The 4D scan is a relatively new development offered by private scanning studios for dads – and mums – who like live-action footage of their unborn child. It's a fabulous 'first' video of your child but not a replacement for routine antenatal scans – and unlike routine scans they can set you back a lot more than the quid the hospital may charge – in some cases 199 times more than that. If you decide to have one, the best time to have a 4D scan is when your partner is between 24 weeks and 30 weeks pregnant. Firms such as www.thisismy.co.uk offer scan packages at locations around the UK.

WHAT TESTS DO DADS HAVE TO TAKE?

Weren't expecting this, were you? The antenatal tests and checks aren't solely the domain of the expectant mother. There's still the small matter of a few prods, jabs and checks that you may need to have. Talk to your GP about the following if you feel they're relevant to you:

A blood-group identifying test

If your partner has a rhesus *negative* blood group but you on the other hand are rhesus *positive* then your baby may be rhesus *positive* too. Because your partner's immune system may treat the baby with the different blood group as an intruder there could be the kind of internal scrap that threatens the life of your baby.

Sickle-cell anaemia

If you've a family history of sickle-cell anaemia you may need to have your blood checked, though you'll only be asked if your partner also has the trait. It's a disease that can cause birth defects and affects people whose families come from Africa, the Caribbean, the Eastern Mediterranean, Middle East and Asia. In Britain sickle-cell is most common in people of African and Caribbean descent (at least 1 in 10–40 have the sickle-cell trait and 1 in 60–200 have sickle-cell disease).

Thalassaemia

Also a type of inherited blood disorder, this can cause anaemia and occurs more frequently in people of Cypriot, Italian, Greek, Indian, Pakistani, Bangladeshi and Chinese descent – this is because the mutations that cause thalassaemia originally occurred in countries in which malaria was common.

Tay-Sachs disease (TSD)

This is very rare in the general population but the defective gene is much more common in people of Ashkenazi (eastern and central European) Jewish descent. TSD is fatal and in order for a child to develop the disease the defective gene must have been passed on from both parents.

Expectancy Explained

Flying Times

Some medical experts advise that pregnant women avoid flying during the first trimester (first 12 weeks of pregnancy). NHS Direct suggest that there's a heightened risk of miscarriage at this time. Talk to your GP or midwife about any travel concerns you may have.

WHAT IF THE SCAN SHOWS TWINS?

Twins, triplets, quadruplets, quins – all right, you get the general idea. OK, the only bad news is that multiple births usually mean you're going to be spending a whole lot more on nappies and baby gear than you would with just one baby. With twins or more your partner may also be advised to rethink her birth plan too. Later in the pregnancy regular checks – including fortnightly scans – may also take place to spot Twin-to-Twin Transfusion Syndrome, which occurs when one twin 'hogs' the placenta and hinders the growth of the other. In the UK, about 1 in every 63 pregnancies results in a multiple birth. There are currently around 12,000 multiple births in the UK each year – and that's a figure that's on the rise, particularly thanks to advances in the areas of infertility and care of premature births. For more information on what happens next, multiple birth issues and discounts on buying more than one buggy, contact the Multiple Births Foundation and the Twins and Multiple Births Association (TAMBA) – see the glossary for details.

4

When Bump Stops the Grind

Pregnancy: Weeks 17-20

The growth of the baby now steps up a pace. Your little boy or girl's body catches up with the head so thankfully everything looks a lot more in proportion. They'll measure around 6½ inches (165mm) at this stage. The facial features become more pronounced and hair begins to grow – they even have their own unique fingerprints. Their eyes grow sensitive to light – in the same way yours will be when they're shining a play torch in your face at 5 a.m. a couple of years from now. Their genitals and reproductive organs are taking shape (that's my boy!) and by the 20th week their skin starts thickening – into four layers – and is covered with a waxy substance called vernix. Vernix moisturises them and stops their skin going the same way your fingers do when you've soaked in the bath too long. It's the reason many babies are born looking a bit, well, like a big ball of cheese. It's OK though, vernix is easily wiped off. Speaking of which – here's the sex stuff.

CAN WE STILL HAVE SEX?

Only around 99.9 per cent of expectant fathers ask this question. Unless you're told otherwise – by the GP or midwife – then there's no reason why you can't both enjoy an active sex life (with each other, of course) virtually throughout the entire pregnancy. Note the word 'virtually' in there, though. There are limits. It's true that sex can be used to help nudge things along when your partner is due to go into labour – a hormone within your semen can kick-start your baby's slide down the birth canal – just don't go at it on the hospital ward. Also be prepared for plenty of disruption to your sex life. Some pregnant women can't get enough sex. In one survey of 17,000 women 36 per cent said their orgasms were more intense when they were pregnant.

Many mothers-to-be switch from one state of sex-hungry nymphomania to the other 'No Way José' frigidity. This even occurs halfway through the act itself. Reasons for this include the changes in hormones and even a sense of feeling sexier about herself (brought on in part by her more ample figure) that is suddenly dampened by concern about the fragile life within her. This mood-swinging attitude to sex isn't unique to her, either.

Some expectant fathers report being even more sexually aroused by their pregnant partner. That's not just because of the physical changes she's undergoing – such as breast engorgement and, er, well, breast engorgement is probably the one that's most caught your eye. Nor is it solely because of the increasingly sexy styles of maternity underwear available to pregnant women these days. (Which, by the way, you can buy her as a gift from such places as www.hotmilklingerie.co.nz or www.figleaves. com – just check on her ever-expanding size before ordering.) No, it's also because of an added emotional element that some men claim raises their desire. Her increased vulnerability can prod some fellas into becoming more sensitive and this, along with the belly rubs or back massages, increases the sense of intimacy between mother- and father-to-be. In short, pregnant couples can get randier.

According to Dr Yvonne K. Fulbright, sex and relationship expert and author of *Your Orgasmic Pregnancy*, the time for things to really start hotting up is from around the 12th week of pregnancy onwards. 'Whether it's her first or second trimester, many women experience increased sexual urges, at levels exceeding pre-pregnancy, but it's during the second trimester in particular, many feel hot to trot for reasons far beyond their control.' Not only that but any anxieties either of you had about getting pregnant will be gone from your mind now too!

Won't sex hurt the baby?

Fear of harming the baby is the number-one reason why many couples go off sex at this time. But unless advised otherwise, it's perfectly safe for couples to enjoy an active sex life throughout the pregnancy, according to Melvyn Dunstall. Just remember that sex during pregnancy comes with a few hidden clauses:

- Things may get uncomfortable, especially for her as she gets bigger – you may need to apply a little imagination to the positions you have sex in.

- You should maintain a sense of humour about things since 'pregnant sex' will often feature odd noises, failed attempts, muscles tensing up or cramp setting in mid-session. Admittedly, even the best stand-up comic may struggle to find much fun in the position you're trying to adopt at this time.

- You're not disturbing the baby. Your nipper is perfectly safe inside its amniotic fluid sac and will not be struck down with a god-awful migraine because of your pounding away.

- Your partner may find that her breasts become sore and overly sensitive – don't be surprised if you're given an order that you can 'look, but don't touch!'

- The use of inanimate objects during sex should be avoided too. (That means vibrators and dildos, not you.) Plastic is a lot less malleable than flesh and in some cases using sex toys could traumatise the placenta.

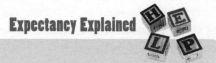

Expectancy Explained

What's Worrying Her . . . An Affair

Some men are afraid of, or even turned off by, the idea of having sex with their partner while she's expecting. It isn't the kind of threesome they had in mind as their ultimate fantasy. Many mothers-to-be feel the same. The fact that they're not getting any sex at home becomes an issue for possibly 10 per cent of expectant fathers who instead seek out sexual satisfaction with someone else. According to relationship psychotherapist Mariam Millar it's a testing time for couples. After all, since you first began trying for a baby you may have enjoyed the most active, regular and at times exciting sex life with your partner you've ever had. Millar suggests that to suddenly change all that once the pregnancy is confirmed is something some men find tough to take.

One US study suggests that during one in every 10 pregnancies the father-to-be has an affair. For some men it could be that they suddenly don't think their woman – when pregnant – is an appropriate sexual partner. Millar believes that in such cases the dad-to-be may be telling himself that fatherhood marks the end of his life as a 'player of the field'. As a result he wants to get one last fling in before the look on his kid's face gives him enough of a guilt complex not to stray any more. In most cases, however, it comes down to sex, or the lack of it. Another survey by www.thebabywebsite.com found that one in 10 pregnant women won't have sex at all once they know they're pregnant – with many opting not to for at least two to three months after it.

The thought of spending up to a year in frustrated denial obviously proves to be too much for some of us.

There are many reasons you may come up with for having an affair while your partner sits at home knitting booties or throwing up but think long and hard about your actions before you do.

As Mariam Millar points out, an affair suggests some serious cracks in your relationship and prompts questions about your commitment to your partner and your role as a father. Consider also the possibly catastrophic repercussions of her finding out that you're playing away while she's carrying your child. At the very least it's hardly a great start to family life.

To avoid going down that route at least talk to her about how you feel. Find out if she just wants to avoid having sex in the early months. See if there are any games you can play or non-penetrative acts you and she can do that'll help you maintain some semblance of a sex life.

Obviously masturbation is an option. But as psychologist Russell Hurn explained to me, your partner can, naturally, feel left out and this act can sometimes isolate people as the man satisfies himself and will then not seek intimacy with the partner. In short, if you can do something sexual together, great – but don't push it. Instead experiment with being intimate without having penetrative sex.

Also remember that she may be very self-conscious about her changing body shape and may not want to expose her body even to someone who's 'seen it all before'. Be tactful, don't make ultimatums or try pointing at your penis and telling her that if you don't use it, you'll lose it.

Talk to your doctor too. Mariam Millar points out that often a basic naivety as to how the human body works makes couples fearful of having sex during pregnancy. Remember, the baby itself is quite well protected in the womb and there's no threat to it from having sex. Be mindful of medical advice, though. Women who've experienced miscarriages in the past may be told by their GP to avoid sex, especially in the first trimester, to reduce any risk of it occurring again.

WHAT ARE THE BEST 'PREGNANT SEX' POSITIONS?

If you and your partner are hoping to keep the bedroom gymnastics flowing for as long as possible during the pregnancy then you're going to have to be flexible, and not just in the Tantric sense either. Sex at this time can still be pretty wild but be prepared for it not necessarily going to plan. Some women find certain positions more comfortable than others and this will change as pregnancy progresses. According to the midwives, there are generally no hard-and-fast rules regarding sex at this time – but avoid rough acts.

It can be common for some vaginal bleeding – or 'spotting' – to occur following sex in pregnancy. It's usually nothing to worry about but if it happens your partner may want to contact the maternity unit for a check. If the whole rigmarole of this expectancy lark has sapped you of your imagination, here's some of the more commonly used – or attempted at least – sex positions for pregnant couples:

Spooning

Aside from the daft name, this position where you lie beside her is a smooth move for you both since it avoids putting pressure on her abdomen and enables you to try positioning yourself behind her at different angles to ease penetration.

Side-by-side

This time you're not putting any weight on her uterus, you're face-to-face and with a bit of leg work – as in crossing your legs over each other's – you're able to penetrate her safely and comfortably.

Her on top

You now get the full view and value of her bump while she gets to 'steer' things a little and can control the depth you go inside her. She can put her hands on your chest to support herself. As she gets heavier you may find that adopting this position with you sat on a chair may work better, as she can take some of her weight on her feet too.

Doggie-style

Particularly practical once her bump gets in the way of almost every other conceivable position – not that conceivable is really an issue any more. Try standing beside the bed while she adopts the all-fours position on it – putting a pillow beneath her belly can make it easier too.

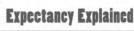

Expectancy Explained

What's Worrying Her – 'I Feel Ugly'

As the hormonal rollercoaster starts to take its toll, she may find she's getting more spots on her face, her skin pigmentation may change – her moles, freckles and nipples get darker – and she may suffer from bleeding gums. She won't like what she's seeing and the way she's feeling at times will only knock her self-esteem even more. The chances are you'll be pretty put off by the whole thing too – but tell her (and reassure yourself) that these changes are temporary. Make an extra effort to tell her how much you love her and find her attractive and how everything is going to be OK. It's traditional at this point to use terms like 'blooming' or in the 'glow of pregnancy' when trying to comfort her. She'll still feel like shit and she may hate you for it but it's a whole lot better than saying stuff like 'gross' right now.

Can oral sex do any harm?

If it's with that girl from the office party it certainly will. Otherwise there's no healthy reason why you and she can't engage in it. There's certainly no truth in the theory that you blowing into her vagina while performing oral sex on her is a dangerous thing to do. Professor Patrick O'Brien blew this myth out of the water for me, explaining that the only real cause for concern when having sex during pregnancy surrounds STIs – sexually transmitted infections. According to O'Brien they can bring on premature labour and cause infection in the baby. If you've got reason to believe you may be bringing home more than just your wage packet while she's pregnant then contact your nearest STI clinic (www.nhs.uk).

HOW SOON AFTER THE BIRTH CAN WE HAVE SEX AGAIN?

It may seem a bit early to be discussing this if you're following this book chronologically, but since we're on the subject anyway we'll look at the options. New mums need time to heal physically and emotionally. Let's face it, if you had just squeezed a basketball out of the end of your penis would you really want to have sex again in a hurry? Sex needs to be slow and gentle and only when she is ready again.

If she had an episiotomy – an incision in the perineum during labour to help deliver the baby – she'll have had internal stitches after the birth and they can take a few weeks to dissolve. Talk things through with her and consider the fact that you'll both be tired and she'll be pretty sore for quite some time after the birth. When the pair of you do get 'back on the bike' then a water-based lubricant like KY Jelly might make things gentler and more bearable. Be aware that breastfeeding mums may find their breasts sore or more sensitive to the touch.

Equally, you may not be so keen on sex at first either. The whole birth process and the trauma involved can leave some men in a state of 'sex shock'. Having seen the more functional side of her body and then breasts in action – or knowing in full, screaming Technicolor what sex can eventually create – can leave you a little less inclined to get back into the routine.

If you are both hot to trot then decide what birth control you're going to use too. Women can conceive as soon as they start to ovulate again – so that's within a month of giving birth. Russell Hurn suggests asking yourselves, 'Do you really want to go through another pregnancy that quickly – having only just stopped fetching bags of sweets from Tesco's at two in the morning?'

BONDING

HOW DO I 'BOND' WITH AN UNBORN BABY?

It can be done – though you're going to have to perform acts of such a seemingly absurd nature to create that perfect bond between father and baby that you may wonder if you're possibly drunk. 'Bonding' has become very big in the world of fatherhood these days. Pregnancy magazines will emphasise the importance of it to your partner – she in turn will have you performing the strangest duties in order for you and the forming foetus to get on like a house on fire.

The popular 'papoose'-style baby carriers serve as something of a metaphor showing how 'new' dads now wear their kids with pride. But the wheels for the bonding process are set in motion many months before you're the one who's carrying the baby.

Of course, not every dad takes to it. For some of us it just doesn't feel natural – for many it's more a case of simply not knowing how to go about it. If you're struggling to 'get into' the pregnancy some of the more common methods dads have used include massaging the bump and putting on some womb music.

How do I massage the bump?

This is a tried and trusted bonding technique for blokes and babies that works on many levels.

First off, the benefits for you: It may be a rare chance for you to enjoy some sensual stroking of the female form at a time when full-on sex is off limits. As a result you see bump rubbing as a means of getting close to your partner. Psychologically it's thought that by doing this you'll lose many of those negative thoughts you have about the baby. You'll grow to love the bump – your child – and realise it's no longer something that's keeping you and your partner apart. Funnily enough there's not much in the way of scientific data backing this up though.

Secondly, with each little kick and movement you get to feel comes a reality check – fatherhood is on its way. According to prenatal massage therapists – yes, such jobs do exist – your touch triggers a chain reaction of stress-relieving happy hormones that has the effect of making your little 'un love you even before it's born.

By massaging your partner's belly you provide gentle muscle relief for her, which in turn leads to the release of 'feel-good' chemicals in her body that the baby enjoys too.

Thirdly, you rubbing oil – massage, not engine – over the bump will release the tension you're feeling too, especially if you've just read the chapter on how much your kid will cost you.

As ever, nothing is definite in pregnancy. You may be excused such happy-clappy chores because some women will establish an exclusion zone around their belly. This is especially true of those mums-to-be who don't want their husbands to see the dark line that mysteriously forms, like a crop circle, running up from their pubic hair to their belly button.

Why the hell should I talk to the bump?

If rubbing her bump felt strange, then this could really freak you out. By just the 16th week of pregnancy your baby's ears are functioning. The ear is one of the earliest organs to fully develop in a baby, so their sense of hearing is one of the first to form. Apparently studies show that from the 24th week onward your baby is listening all the time. So keep the swearing down and turn the iPod up.

EXPECTANT DADS' EXPERIENCES

Bonding with the Bump

'I would play my Northern Soul records when my wife Lisa was pregnant with our baby, Julia. Sure enough, after Julia was born she'd calm down to my music when I played it in her room.'

Richard F

'The thing that made it real for me was listening to the little thing move inside my wife's belly.'

Dominic N

'For the final three months of my wife Helen's pregnancy I would read Magic Roundabout books to her bulging belly each night. We were keen to try anything that would give our son Eddy a good start in life. I can't say for sure if it's made him a cleverer child or if he responded to my voice more because I'd been droning on about Dylan and Zebedee for the final trimester – but I still enjoy reading to him now.'   Matt B

Research shows that the more you talk to the bump – yes, talk – or even sing to it, the more your baby will hear. Just reading the sports pages from the newspaper out loud can help a child recognise his or her father's voice, according to Dunstall. If nothing else you could be sowing the seeds of football team allegiance – or familiarising your kid with your team's rubbish form – from a very early age.

Did you know?

Voice Recognition

In tests newborn babies are more responsive to a familiar voice, turning their head to a voice they 'recognise' as opposed to one they don't on 80 per cent of occasions.

HOW CAN I GET INTERESTED IN THE WHOLE PREGNANCY LARK?

As much as you may want to be a part of the occasion, it's easy for fathers to feel left out of what's happening. If the idea of belly rubbing or talking to her navel leaves you cold there are other things you can do with your partner that can help reinforce the bond between father and unborn child. Such as:

Attending the scans

'The minute I saw our daughter on the ultrasound scan I'd say we started to bond, I could see her tiny hand and hear her tiny heart beating – it was fuzzy but it was the most beautiful thing I'd ever seen,' says expectant dad John L. Keep the image from the scan with you – in your wallet or as your desktop wallpaper – and make it a talking point.

Take on a project

If the scan hasn't left you gushing then maybe a more functional involvement in the pregnancy could help build a link between you and your baby. 'The first thing my wife did was buy *me* a baby book,' explains Charley G. 'During the pregnancy I was in charge of sticking in the scan pictures, the significant events and recording her statistics and feelings.'

Become an expert

Read up on the birth, your role and what your partner's going through. OK, obviously by reading this you are – but take a look at some of the literature she's reading. Pregnancy magazines can be insightful – not just the lingerie section – and helpful in getting you focused on things. Look online too.

Test yourself

One game I played when my wife was expecting that helped me get into the 'birth spirit' was Pregnancy Pub Quiz. I would start browsing her magazines and then she'd test me! You get familiar with the terminology of pregnancy and feel you have a little more understanding of and control over what's going on. I didn't get any prizes but the information sank in and I knew our birth plan better than I did the list of FA Cup winners since 1980 by the end of it.

Practical Matters

Pregnancy: Weeks 21-24

By week 20 your baby will be sleeping, dreaming and waking up. Your partner should have a noticeable bump by now – you could be sprouting one yourself – while inside little junior will be moving around and will now be able to hear sounds outside the womb. It'll weigh around 1½lb (680g). She could even start experiencing Braxton Hicks contractions – false ones – 'twinges' that are preparing her uterus for the birth.

Expectancy Explained

The Twenty-week Scan

This is also called the anomaly scan; it's when you can find out the sex of your baby, get a picture of it, see its limbs and head, as well as learning crucial information about its health. The size and shape of your baby's heart – even the workings of the heart valves – are checked at this point. The sonographer will be able to see that organs such as the kidneys are developing OK. They'll also be able to tell whereabouts the baby's feeding sac – the placenta – is positioned. If the sonographer thinks something needs double-checking they will tell you to arrange another scan with an obstetrician within the next three days.

EXPECTANT DADS' EXPERIENCES

Finding Out the Baby's Sex

'We didn't want to know the sex of our baby. The great thing is that neither of us has a feeling of what it is and we both want a boy or a girl so to be kept guessing for all this time has been fun. There are so few real surprises these days.'   Matthew D

'I initially felt it would have been better not to know the sex of the baby to stop people from buying lots of blue or pink stuff for us, but knowing has made it easier. Especially to focus on name choosing, which is difficult.'   Tom L

'Sarah was not sure but it seemed illogical to me not to know. You need to buy stuff up front, and sex is important to what you buy and what you do with the nursery. People have said that it will take away from the surprise on the day – I can't see what possible difference it could make. Holding my baby for the first time is going to be such a moment that I don't think that I will give a monkey's about the sex. In fact knowing the sex earlier is possibly marginally helpful – however you look at it, most parents (I would imagine) initially have a preference for either a boy or a girl. I'm not sure that I wouldn't feel a little guilty if I had been hoping one way and it turned out the other on the day. Knowing in advance means that this is not even a consideration on the day.'   Dominic N

'We did find out that we are having a boy. Finding out allowed us to change from thinking about having a pregnancy to focusing on having a baby. This was important to us partly because the pregnancy wasn't planned. We had no preference for a boy or girl and this made it easier. Having a new baby will be

enough of a surprise – finding out the sex of the baby couldn't add to that.'
                                                                    Charley G

WHAT DO WE DO AFTER THE SCAN?

Once you're clear of those stages in the pregnancy where there's the greatest risk of miscarriage and your partner is well into her second trimester, then dads-to-be can start getting down and dirty with the more practical, physical elements of pregnancy. You get to release your inner hunter-gatherer.

It's time to start planning the nursery, organising your budget for when your partner's income drops, moving house if you need to, or changing the car at least. You should start window-shopping at least for essential items for your baby – like its bed and buggy – and also learn how to avoid the marketing traps designed to extract the precious pennies from a pregnant couple.

It may still seem like early days to be worrying about this but there are a number of reasons why now is the best time to get started with these projects:

Firstly, your partner is still able to actively help out with stuff around the house if you're decorating or moving – she won't be for much longer.

Secondly, it will focus your mind too. As psychologist Russell Hurn observes, as your partner gets bigger and the impact of the pregnancy starts to take hold on you, then you can experience some anxiety. By getting hands-on with the buying and nest building you feel as if you're playing a useful role and are in some ways prepared for the big change coming your way.

Thirdly – and this is a rare one but worth considering anyway – it's not impossible that your baby could be born premature, even as early as 24 weeks. The more you can prepare for now, the easier it'll be when the baby does arrive.

Did you know?

Weight and See

Your partner will put on between and 22 and 28lb (10–12kg) during pregnancy. The bulk (don't use this word in her company) of this will occur from the 20th week onwards. It won't all be baby making up that weight either, thankfully for her, since a 28lb baby would bring tears to anyone's eyes. The areas where she'll 'pad out' a little include her all-over body size, due to the 4lb in additional fluid flowing around her body (especially her ankles), 1.5lb worth of placenta (the baby's 'food' in the womb) and 2lb in extra breast size.

SHOULD WE MOVE HOUSE TO MAKE ROOM FOR THE NEW ARRIVAL?

If things didn't sound like one hell of a stress-filled headache already, then here's another quandary for you. Becoming a parent is definitely up there in that list of the most traumatic things you'll do in life. So is moving house. Why would anyone in their right mind even consider doing both at the same time?

Your first child is most likely to come along while you and your partner are still living in the first home you got together, when one of you 'shacked up' with the other or when you both took the leap on to the property ladder. At the time the only extra space you needed was for drunken friends sleeping over on the sofa. Now things have changed. Now you're going to have to devote an entire room of your home to someone who will only get bigger and bigger and – as only humans and magpies do – will accumulate more shiny junk the older they get.

Only you know for sure how your current home will hold up to your new arrival. But don't panic about getting a bigger home. After all, for the first six months after the birth you'll probably have your baby sleeping in your room with you – he or she won't be crawling around until later than that, by which point you'll have got the gist of folding down that buggy to save space too. But if you are going to do it then here are some of the experiences of fathers who've gone before:

Earlier in the pregnancy is better

Your partner will be able to do more and cope with the whole thing a little easier and you'll have more energy than you will if she's at 38 weeks and tossing and turning all night. Plus you'll have fewer items to pack since it's unlikely that you'll have bought a lot of gear in the early months.

But don't fret if you can't do it straight away

'When we moved, Helen was five months pregnant,' says Matt B, father of Eddy, George and Alice. 'In a way that was good because there was less risk of the stress affecting the baby and equally she wasn't busting for a pee all the time.'

Pack now

Put the non-essential stuff in boxes as soon as you know you're moving and just keep the day-to-day stuff out. 'Once the baby arrives you're not going to have the time or inclination to unpack everything, so if there's stuff you can store away for months, do it,' says Matt.

Get home help

Friends or removal firms that will pack and unpack for you could prove to be a worthwhile added expense at this stage, if you can afford to do it. Don't be afraid to shop around and ask for discounts. Some firms will pack and unpack for you for nothing if they're going to get your business.

Be prepared for chaos

'In the end it took about a year for us to finally settle in to our new house,' says Matt B. 'If you can, get one room unpacked and as comfortable as you can and then do the next.'

Stay with friends and family

Don't be afraid to call upon relatives as a place to stay while the move is going on or if the house you're moving into is in need of some work. If you're going to be without a kitchen for a month or two it's better that your partner at least stays somewhere with all the facilities she needs, even if it means spending some time apart.

Think about safety

That's not a call to go around covering the plug sockets and locking the bleach cupboard – though you will need to do that once your child is on the move. Just be sure to contact the nearest hospital to your new home and ensure your partner registers with a local GP as soon as possible. Think about the place you're moving to and how your partner will cope there once she's at home alone with the baby. Are there a lot of stairs? Will it be easy getting a pram in and out?

Why are we talking about schools already?

Even though your child has yet to be born, the subject of which school he or she will be going to is something that, believe it or not, you will get asked about. Not without good reason, either. If you live near a church that sponsors or is in some way linked to a particularly good school – good exam results, high Ofsted rating, it's not a smouldering ruin – then you'll probably already be aware of the effect this has upon new parents within your local area.

As a YouGov 2008 revealed – despite plummeting house prices at the time – one in three parents still admitted to being prepared to spend more than £50,000 extra on a home just to get their kids into the best state schools. This is the world you're now entering. New parents eager to get their kids into a 'model' church school will move house, drive to another parish from miles away, usurp ageing relatives or convert religion with no qualms whatsoever. Talking to some people you may feel that your child's name should be put down on a school's waiting list before the ink's even dried on the birth certificate, or you've actually settled on a name!

The same YouGov study into state schools found that one in five parents would be prepared to commute further to work and 12 per cent would move away from friends and family if it meant that their home was close to a better school. The survey also found that a third of parents said that the quality of schools in an area would play a big part in their decision to buy a house. If you're considering it then you're not alone in doing so. In many cases pre-school nurseries – your child's first step on the education ladder, which can begin from three years old – are linked to local infant schools. Getting your child into these schools may prove easier if they've already attended the attached nursery, though this isn't a certainty.

Where you live in respect to a school's catchment area will have a major bearing on your child's chances of being given a place at the school you eventually want them to attend. Before you move contact the local authority in your chosen area and check out which schools/nurseries fall into which catchment areas.

BUYING BABY GEAR

HOW MUCH IS OUR BABY GOING TO COST US?

Every few months a scare story appears in the papers about how much it costs to raise a kid in the UK these days. The frightening figures these stories throw up – the Centre for Economics and Business Research claims a baby born in 2016 would cost £231,843 by the age of 21 – are used by firms with something to plug. That something is usually a financial service designed to ease the cost of having a kid. Look into the small print of these tales and you can see how such ludicrous figures might occur – if you're heading off to Disneyland every half-term, leaving your kid with a private nanny for 12 hours a day and upgrading from a moped to a Humvee then yes, your child will be said to be very expensive. In truth, having a baby won't bankrupt you – but you will have to take a closer interest in your incomes and outgoings.

Your income will most likely drop while your partner is out of work or on maternity leave and you'll need to prepare for that. Also you'll spend more on your child from way before it is born – and possibly a lot less on the luxuries you've enjoyed up until now too.

But equally both your partner and you will be eligible for financial support in a number of forms. You'll also start enjoying many of the family discount deals available on everything from days out to restaurant dinners and for the first couple of months you won't be able to move for gifts from friends, hand-me-downs from relatives and, if you're on the right mailing list, freebies from baby-gear firms.

So the headlines you see, like 'Cost of Raising Kids Soars', should be treated the same way your newborn child would treat them when they reach around six months old: grab them, chew them, realise they're worthless and not tasty, and then spit them out.

The cost of your new kid will weigh heavy on your mind throughout the pregnancy and for at least the next 20 years probably. There will, of course, be things your new baby will need. But equally there's a lot of stuff marketed at new parents that you'll either use sparingly or else will simply gather dust while the rest of your purchases are being covered with sick, food and wee.

You and your partner will spend the next six months at least arguing as to which bits you should buy as new, which items you're better off asking others to buy as gifts and what stuff you should be bidding for online or shunning altogether. A few basics for you to consider are:

WHERE SHOULD WE BUY NEW BABY GEAR?

You're spoiled for choice these days. Mothercare no longer corners the market in sprog-wear and accessories – though they're still an ideal under-one-roof starting point and a good place to send friends and relatives who are keen to buy gifts.

The growth in online shopping certainly hasn't passed the world of baby bits and bobs by either. Everything from eco-friendly nappies to DIY Doppler foetal scans can be purchased via Google – often saving you money and a Saturday-morning schlep in the process. As a result, links to useful websites are provided throughout this section – be sure to check out parenting websites for bargain deals too.

WHAT DO WE ACTUALLY NEED TO BUY FOR OUR BABY?

It may seem as if you're being pressured into buying a mountain of unnecessary add-ons for your baby – and that's just by your missus – but there are a number of 'essentials' that it would be pretty tough for you to raise your baby without. Your budget and the generosity of friends and relatives will help determine what stuff you have, but if you're looking to prioritise your spending here's a rundown of the gear to get and a range of prices you could pay for them – so get your calculator out and pour yourself a stiff drink.

These prices were sourced at the time of going to print and are intended to give you an idea of what you can pay in order to plan your budget.

Before you start looking, try setting yourselves an amount you're going to spend on the accessories and make sure you shop around – if nothing else, wandering around the baby section of John Lewis is all part of the bonding process too.

Moses baskets

Particularly useful as your new baby's chief form of sleeping arrangement for the first couple of months, although it'll face stiff competition from your partner's breast or even your chest. Since your baby may well be sleeping in the same room as you for the first six months, a Moses basket can be an ideal bed if space is tight too. The baskets are carried, well, basket-style really, then parked on a separate 'collapsible' stand. The word collapsible doesn't feel right when talking about a baby's sleeping arrangements, does it?

From around: £38 (www.mothercare.com) or as little as £2 (starting bid) for a used one on eBay.

Bassinet or crib

Instead of the basket some parents opt for a more rigid crib or bassinet bed for their baby (usually after reading the word 'collapsible' in the previous paragraph). Rocking cribs can be especially good for getting your nipper off to sleep – the rocking and the motion has a calming effect. On the down side these aren't as portable as a Moses basket, which your partner may want to carry around the house during the day when she's home alone. The temptation to simply stick the kid in bed with you to sleep for now should be resisted, not only on the grounds of safety – they need a controlled temperature and no 15-stone men rolling on top of them (see more on this in Chapter 11) – but also because babies love nothing more than getting into a routine and your sex life has been interrupted enough by them before they were born.

From around: £129 Boori Urban Bassinet (mothercare.com).

Cot bed

Possibly the best idea of the lot if you're on a budget. These are built to last your child from day one until they're five years old. As they get older you simply remove the bars and upgrade any 'extras' from early years 'Beatrix Potter bunny mobiles' to toddler time Ben 10 or Angelina Ballerina bedspread and pillowcases. Again you can get a decent second-hand cot bed – just be sure to clean it up, use a non-toxic paint if you're changing its colour to suit the nursery décor, and always replace any missing or broken bars and make sure the sides slide and lock safely. Then simply add a new mattress, which will set you back around £20.

From around: £99 for an Ashton Cot Bed up to the Humphrey Cot Bed £270 (both www.mothercare.com), or a Mothercare three-stage cot bed advertised on www.gumtree.com for £65.

Changing table

Some changing tables aren't much more than flat boards that can fit over a cot – others come in the form of a full-on chest of drawers with an oversized top surface area on which you plonk your baby to change their nappy, dress them and do things like apply baby cream. Of course, you can use the floor to do all this. (It's a safer option too, since holding your baby in place three or four feet above the ground with one hand while rifling through drawers for nappies or baby wipes certainly isn't a move straight from the midwives' handbook.) On the plus side the changing table will save you a lot of backache as you're able to change your baby at waist level, not hunched over on the floor. It'll also double as decent storage space for their room for a good few years – just avoid putting any shelves above it if you value your own skull.

From around: £63 for a trolley-style Ella table to £299 for a Boori Sleigh changer (www.johnlewis.com), or an Ikea table from £15 on eBay.

Bedding

Baby sleeping bags are a popular and safe option – there's no worrying about them pulling these over their head as they might with a loose blanket. Duvets and pillows are not recommended for your baby until he or she is a year old because they can restrict your baby's movement and may make them too hot. For safety reasons avoid putting soft toys in the cot too.

From around: £20.50 for a baby sleeping Grobag at www.gro.co.uk.

Mobiles

Not an early introduction into the world of text messaging, but a moving, soothing mobile that dangles over the cot and hypnotises your newborn. Colourful, musical ones keep your kid surprisingly entertained in the early days when they have the recall of a goldfish.

From around: £34 Happy Safari musical mobile (www.elc. co.uk) – this one was also seen on eBay with starting bids of £2.

Baby bath

Babies love a dip in the tub almost as much as a pair of consenting adults, and you can go from using a bowl at first, to a simple plastic tub or moulded bath, right through to a specially designed non-slip mat – called an Aquapod – that supports your baby once it can sit up in the bath (from about six months). Alternatively you could just wash them in the sink or shower with you until they're old enough to be embarrassed by it. (See 'How Do I Bathe Our Baby?', Chapter 11.)

From around: £7.99 Little Fish Baby Bath (www.mothercare. com).

Clothes/body suits

From the moment they're born your baby will shoot through these. You should get at least half a dozen to use and wash in the first week. Little cardigans and a winter suit are a must too. These are usually gender-specific and often have fun patterns, characters or football team crests on them – and most of all they're cheap. As a result friends and relatives will buy them for your child by the bulk load. Ideally go for white, 100 per cent cotton versions.

From around: £7 for a pack of 5 (www.johnlewis.com).

Nappies

A must. Babies produce an unfeasible amount of waste and these are the best way to deal with it. The type you use will depend upon whether you and your partner want to use disposable or reuseable (previously called terry or washable) ones. Both have an effect on the environment – the relative impact of dumping or washing nappies is a topic of much debate – and both will hit you in the pocket, although in the case of reuseables only once. Babies need to be changed, on average, 10 times a day (which gradually reduces as they grow), and at each change they need wiping up and the disposable nappies need to be binned. Many choose to use scented bags for this task, though you could consider the planet a little and just fold and seal the nappy before throwing it away.

So you'll need to buy baby wipes and bags on a regular basis too. Several studies suggest that using disposable nappies throughout the entire time until a baby is potty trained (usually around two and a half years old) will set you back on average £1,200 to £1,500 – reuseable ones are estimated to come in at around £350 to £700 over a 30-month period, including your laundry costs. Extras with the reuseable ones include disposable liners and a storage bucket. However, these are based on averages. Your baby may need more changes or fewer. Your choice of which nappies you use may change according to what's available at the time, and you can get washable wipes instead of disposable ones, which will affect the cost too. One thing's guaranteed. You will need to use something.

From around: £3.75 Tesco Loves Baby Ultra Dry Size 5 Economy Pack 40.

Changing bag and changing mat

You and your partner may already have a baggage collection that's on a par with Heathrow but these purpose-built, multi-pocketed numbers are a real plus. There's also a range of fashionable, record-carrier-style versions for chaps too. Rapidly moving up alongside the baby carrier as the 'modern dad' badge of honour, these bags are a lot more image-friendly for the dads to carry than Mum's changing bags. Classier than ramming everything in a plastic carrier bag too. Also, your vocabulary will be enriched with the term 'muslin' cloth. These will be used to wipe up all your baby discharges when feeding – they cost next to nothing but are worth their weight in congealed baby vomit for sure.

From around: £29.95 Tintamar VIP 2 Dadbag (www.happy-bags.co.uk), Skötsam babycare mat, Ikea £5.

Bottles and steriliser

With the best will in the world there's every chance your partner will give up the ghost with breastfeeding within a month or two of your baby being born. She'll be complaining of aching nipples or just be too knackered to carry on – in some cases she'll not be able to provide enough milk as your ravenous offspring develops a thirst that suggests he or she is a real chip off the old block. Fortunately formula milk is a safe option; the kids certainly seem to like it and you can keep it as sterile as breast milk by using a steam cleaning device or one that cleans the bottles on a hot spin in the microwave.

From around: Avent Express Steam 6 Bottle Steriliser – £26, Boots.com.

Baby monitor

You can get versions that double as temperature gauges, ones with built-in video cameras, and many walkie-talkie types even clip on to your belt in case you spend most nights aimlessly wandering around the rooms of your own home wondering how you got into this mess. There's a roaring baby monitor market on eBay since they're virtually redundant within a few weeks of your baby being born. Many parents just find the constant vigil of watching it – and the resultant paranoia caused by your baby deviously holding its breath – too much to handle.

Others realise that they're only ideal for listening to their partner talking to themselves, breaking wind or slagging them off while they're in the baby's room. Some have discovered that these monitors come into their own when you take your baby away to a hotel with you – ideally a hotel with thin walls and a decent bar.

From around: £32, BT Digital Baby Monitor 300 (John Lewis).

Beg, Borrow or Steal Items

Once you've told the world you're about to become a dad, be sure to tap up any fathers you know for the following bits of kit. These are items you'll need further down the line, when your baby is moving of its own accord. Any dad with grown-up kids will have these, gathering dust in attics or the backs of drawers somewhere. They cost almost nothing brand new but second-hand they act as a token of 'bonding' among dads. Your mate may not have any sound advice on raising kids – but he's a great source of the following:

- **Electrical socket covers** – plastic socket plugs that stop toddlers fingering themselves into the national grid.
- **Cupboard locks** – screw-on clips that make the door to the cabinet beneath the sink out of bounds to all but the most dexterous of adults.
- **Toilet seat lock** – similar clip-style arrangement that will stop your toddler tossing your iPhone/wallet/cat down the lav.
- **Corner guards** – plastic protectors that will ease the impact of your toddler's head against coffee table, wooden chair, TV unit, cupboard corner etc., etc. The list, as both you and your local A&E will discover, is endless.

WHY SO MANY BUGGIES AND WHICH ONE SHOULD WE BUY?

Just like cars, there's a baby buggy to fit every pocket, every taste, every lifestyle and every desire to outdo the person next to you at the traffic lights. At first your baby will simply lie there, snoozing away, while you take them on tour – but within six months they'll be sat bolt-upright like a *Strictly Come Dancing* judge, gripping the safety bar and eagerly eyeing up everything. Bear this in mind when choosing your buggy. Some parents opt for a traditional-style pram at first and then find they have to buy a separate buggy or stroller further down the line. Since babies have to lie flat at first then traditional prams or 'suitable from birth' buggies are the ones to go for. Usually cost and personal taste are the deal breakers but there are a number of often-overlooked factors you need to consider to avoid buying a dud.

Buy the buggy before the birth

If you're going to be taking your newborn baby home from hospital in your own car then it may be wise to have bought your buggy or travel system before the birth, since these often come with a baby seat designed to fit in most cars. The Travel System form combines the buggy/pushchair with a removable carrier that doubles as a car seat – it's especially handy if you're restricted when it comes to space at home, since it also acts as a transportable day cot that takes up less space than a Moses basket.

Buggies can screw your back up

What may suit your partner may not suit you. You should both try pushing the buggy in the store before buying – ideally with it adjusted to a height you're both comfortable with. Expectant fathers need to watch to make sure there's sufficient distance between your step as you walk and the back axles of the buggy. It should accommodate your natural stride. Seriously! It may sound like a bit of papa pampering here, but according to a survey by BackCare – the charity for healthier backs – poor pushchair-pushing posture not only makes for a great tongue twister but also accounts for back pain in an estimated 73 per cent of new parents! Perfect your pushing technique, get comfy with the buggy and learn how to adjust it easily and safely before buying.

Buggies have 'a knack'

'There's a knack to this' is the line you'll hear used again and again by exasperated fathers and confused shop-floor demonstrators whenever they're trying to fold down a new buggy. It usually ends up with both, plus one other assistant, ganging up in a scene reminiscent of a pack of wild dogs dragging down a flailing water buffalo. But you and your partner will often be alone trying to dismantle the buggy – in many cases one-handed, since you'll be clutching your child in the other. Practise doing it in the store several times and at home many more and, if push really comes to shove, stoop to reading the instruction manual.

Buggies don't fit every car boot

Some stores may let you take a buggy down to the car park, fold it down and see if it'll stash away safely in the boot of your car. These stores exist only in your dreams so, ideally, measure the height, width and depth of your boot – then do the same with the buggy.

Buggies can be urban or off-road

OK, they're not marketed as such, but do think about how and where you live before buying your wheels. Some are incredibly sturdy-looking 'tankers' with baskets in the undercarriage and wheels like a tractor's. Great for outward bounders, but a real wrestle for getting on buses. Others are featherlight, minimalist designs that prove to be ideal for busy urban environments and stairs – but they can easily make an image-wary male look as if he's mooching around with a drinks trolley. If you're very much an outdoorsy couple then some buggies enable you to run or jog with your baby too – see www.mountainbuggy.com.

EXPECTANT DADS' EXPERIENCES

Buying Buggies

'We went with a Bugaboo. I bought it through Mothercare – they have an online discount code for 10 per cent, which seems to change every year but if you search round the blogs you can find it. I wanted it to last a few years and with this you can detach all the fabric and throw it in the washing machine – which will help its sell-on value too.'
Dominic N

'For us it was a lightweight stroller that we tried out in John Lewis but bought – for less – off a website we'd never heard of. We needed one that would be easy to get on and off public transport, we didn't need the extras like a car seat, though I'd have liked a three-wheeler to be able to go on bumpier walks, but they were all too big and heavy for Sarah.'
Charley G

'Don't scrimp on this one, it's important to make sure your wife is able to get out and about as soon as possible and the

*buggy can make or break that. Mel started going for walks
with the baby in the first week, which kept her happy and
meant I came home to a happy household.'* Matthew D

How much will the buggy cost?

Again, you can go for the second-hand option and save yourself
some serious expense on this item. The price will vary according
to the make, the type and any extras you may need. Here's a
quick rundown of the various styles with a rough price indicator
guide for brand-new ones:

- **3-in-1 combinations**
  Shaped like a pram but can convert into a pushchair that
  faces forward or rearward. Example: Concord Neo
  Mobility (including 0 Group car seat, rain cover and para-
  sol), £599.99.

- **Travel systems**
  Featuring removable car seat that doubles as a carrier for
  shipping your kid around the home too. Pushchair chassis
  and basket for carrying spares (accessories, not spare
  babies). Example: Graco Quattro Tour Travel System,
  £251.99.

- **Three-wheelers**
  Ignore the connotations of Del Boy and naff yellow
  cars; these nippy designs are sturdy enough and
  especially good for tricky corners and going over bumpy
  terrain, since many have air tyres instead of hard plastic
  wheels – which may make your baby's ride a little
  smoother. On the down side they can get punctures.
  Example: Quinny Buzz Xtra Pushchair Silver/Rocking
  Black £359.95.

- **Pushchairs/Strollers**
Forward-facing design with storage basket underneath, these are especially easy to fold and very lightweight, so ideal for parents using public transport a lot. Example: Maclaren Techno XT, £220.00.

Did you know?

The Way a Buggy Faces Can Influence Your Child's Reading Skills

Recent research from the University of Dundee shows that babies who are pushed in prams or buggies that face the parent, rather than face away, are less stressed. Dads are also twice as likely to speak to their baby when they're in a buggy facing them – which the researchers found made babies more likely to laugh and more self-aware.

Make a Buggy-buying Check-list

Make a note of the following when road-testing your kid's carriage:

- Can you adjust the handle height so that a tall dad can use it without stooping?
- How easy is it to collapse down – both try doing it. Then borrow a wriggling, wailing, 10lb baby from someone and try doing it one-handed.
- Can you apply and release the brakes easily?
- Does it feel secure and is it easy to clean?
- Will it fit in your car boot? On the bus? In your home?

Expectancy Explained HELP

Prepare to be Junk Dumped

Events like the Baby Show (www.thebabyshow.co.uk) held at the Birmingham NEC among other venues nationwide are great places for comparing the wide world of baby gear in one long trudge. On the plus side you get to see what's on offer, you get free promotional goodies, you get ideas for the nursery and both you and your partner get a taster of how your life is about to change as you mingle with other prospective wide-eyed young mums and tight-arsed young dads. However, the firms flogging their wares at these shows do also deluge you with online offers and junk mail the moment you get home. Admittedly, you could get some freebies out of anything you sign up for on the day – but be prepared for the sales stalking that will follow for months and years to come.

WHAT ABOUT THE CAR SEAT?

There's no gender split when it comes to buying baby stuff; certainly the vendor doesn't seem to care who taps in the PIN when you're buying a pushchair with a name like a marsupial or Elizabethan slang that costs more than your car's worth.

However, leaving the Bugaboos and Quinnys aside, there are some purchases that dads almost have a paternal duty to play a part in. To make things easier when it comes to stocking up on stuff for the baby, the pair of you could devise a list of things to research and buy and then split it. But if you're the one who does most of the driving – or you're simply very precious about your car – you may want to make the buying of the car seat daddy domain.

You can get car seats from high street outlets such as Halfords, Mothercare and the John Lewis Partnership – or online through websites belonging to the major brands such as Britax, Graco and Maxi Cosi. It's a good idea to compare prices. The same goes for other heavy-duty – and heavy-outlay – items such as buggies, sleep monitors (you can get either audio or digital video ones to give your child an early introduction to a life of CCTV surveillance) and cot beds.

Buying a seat from the high street store allows you to manhandle the goods and there should be a specialist expert on hand to show you how to fit it and point out the various extras or differences between the styles.

If you're going to be taking your baby home by car from the hospital after it's born then you must have a child car seat for them. The law in the UK dictates that kids today must use some form of car seat or booster from birth up to the age of 12.

But if you're not buying a seat until after the baby arrives then many larger stores – including Mothercare – provide a 'test dummy' seat. You can plonk your baby in, gauge the size, get used to the straps and generally get a feel for how these things work.

At this point – 20-odd weeks into the pregnancy – you may still be thinking about budgets and prices. The leading brands to look at when drawing up your budget include:

Car seats:
- Bebe Confort www.bebeconfort.com
- Britax www.britax.co.uk
- Graco www.graco.co.uk
- Maxi-Cosi www.maxi-cosi.com
- Mamas and Papas www.mamasandpapas.com

Pushchairs:

- Bugaboo www.bugaboo.com
- Chicco www.chicco.co.uk
- Graco www.graco.co.uk
- Maclaren www.maclarenbaby.com
- Mothercare www.mothercare.com
- Quinny www.quinny.com

What am I looking for when buying the baby's car seat?

As tempting as it is in these cash-strapped times to go second-hand on these more pricy purchases – it's advisable that you don't skimp on the car seat.

'You really want to know the provenance on safety items like the car seat,' explains Guy Bird, a motoring journalist and father of two who regularly road-tests family cars for *FQ* magazine. According to the Royal Society for the Prevention of Accidents (RoSPA) this is in case there's a hidden fault with the seat or its been damaged in an accident. So avoid buying one you don't know the history of – but do consider it if trusted friends offer you a perfectly sound one gathering dust in their attic.

With a child on the way you should be looking for a rear-facing Group 0 car seat. This should keep your kid safe and sound from birth up until nine months – when they weigh up to 9kg (20lb) and are able to sit up unaided and support their head on their own.

You can get group 0+ from birth up to 13kg (28lb), which is around 15 to 18 months.

If you're after something that will last longer then consider models such as the Britax First Class, which is a seat suitable from birth to four years (up to 18kg, or 40lb). It can be used rearward facing up to 13kg and then forward facing for 9 to 18kg.

Your baby son or daughter's first 'optional extra' could be a car sunshade. Yes, even in the UK you'll need it one day. You can get smiley-face ones that stick on the windscreen and keep your baby protected from the sun's rays. Or, if you're already seething at having to deface your motor with a 'Baby on Board' sticker, then opt for the roller-blind type.

Will the seat fit my car?

If your car was manufactured after 1999 it should come with ISOFIX – International Standards Organisation Fix – anchors either side of the cushion in the rear passenger seat. These fix in to the chassis of the car. This is a much more secure way than simply running an adult seat belt through the slots on some car seats, according to Guy Bird.

But car seats, seat belts and these anchorage points can vary between different models of cars. As a result it's pretty tough trying to find a seat that fits all cars, and while the ISOFIX points are designed to get around this, some models of car only take some types of ISOFIX seat. To see which seat will fit your car, check your car manufacturer's website – compatible models should be listed.

If they're not or if you're not sure about the seat you're looking to buy, then go to a specialist store. Halfords have dedicated car-seat people on hand to run you through the types of car seats available and help you fit them securely.

If you're purchasing a travel system – a combination buggy and car seat – again have a store expert show you how it fits in your car before you buy it.

If you're going to be driving with your child pretty regularly throughout its first year or so – possibly dropping them with baby minders – then be sure to check out the seats that come with separate base models. Here the base clips into the car's ISOFIX points, then the seat itself secures into the base. They're just as secure, but once fitted you don't have to remove the whole seat frame every time you take your baby out of the car. You simply click the seat back into place each journey.

If you're expecting twins, then definitely point this out to the likes of Halfords, who offer discounts on 'bulk' buys – as well as viewing the range on offer with the Twins and Multiple Birth Association. For more advice on problems with car seats check out www.childcarseats.org.uk.

Tips for Taking Baby by Car

- Fit your baby's seat so he or she is sat behind you – your partner can sit behind the passenger seat if she's travelling in the back or can turn around to check on baby if she's in the front.
- Get a mini-mirror that sticks to the inside of the rear windscreen. Angle it so you can see your baby in this mirror when you look into your rear-view mirror.
- If the fittings allow, put a plastic sheet under the car seat or base to keep any food, milk, crumbs and much worse off the upholstery.
- Get into the habit of keeping a kid's bag in the boot – stocked with toys, books and a spare blanket.
- Once your kid is old enough for a forward-facing seat – size Group 1 for kids weighing around 9kg (20lb), at about 12 months old – then also fit a protective cover to the back of your seat. Muddy wellies won't do the upholstery on the back of your seat any favours.

HOW DO I AVOID BEING RIPPED OFF BUYING BABY GEAR?

Since baby accessories don't really suffer much in the way of wear and tear – mainly because your kid will grow out of things before you've even had the credit card bill for them arrive – you can pick up plenty of very-good-condition, second-hand gear. It's a practical solution at a time when your finances can be especially tight and a sure-fire way of not paying over the odds for stuff you'll soon be done with.

But it can jar with your desire (OK, her demands) to get the very best for your new baby. Be prepared for some conflict here, since expectant mothers foster a competitive spirit that puts most alpha males to shame when it comes to babies. If you are agreed on trying to save some cash – and not too fussed about junior being decked out in this month's latest baby designer labels – then the best sources for gear are:

'Nearly-new' baby sales

That's second-hand to you and me. There's no shame in picking up almost pristine baby grows, booties or even a buggy for as little as to a tenth of the original cost. These sales are arranged by the National Childbirth Trust, a support charity for new parents, and feature everything from prams and toys to changing mats and clothes. Once you've drawn up your list of essentials and made a rough estimate of the prices you'll pay for new stuff, then seek out the next nearly-new sale in your area. As a rule of thumb look to pay no more than a third of the original cost of any items you're after. Go to the NCT website (http://www.nct.org.uk/in-your-area/event-finder), tap in your postcode and find out when and where the next jumble-sale-style new parents gathering will be.

eBay/Gumtree/Preloved

Admittedly you're buying stuff as seen in a thumbnail picture that tells you more about the seller's poor taste in home décor than it does the actual product – but the online auction site is still a useful place to save some cash when nest building. At the time of writing an expectant dad on eBay could pick up a Tomy Baby Monitor that would retail for £40 as new for just £8. There was a double-seated pushchair (for twins) that would have been £220 on offer for just £50 and a BabyDan changing unit that sold for new at £220 – up for grabs at bids starting from £4.99! On the down side, you'd have to go and collect it – but with the money you'd saved elsewhere, you could hire a limo to do that. Best of all, Freecycle.org is an online community where people offer unwanted stuff for free in a bid to recycle toys, baby clothes, etc.

Comparison and mother-and-baby websites

Another bonus side to the internet for expectant fathers (there are many, but we won't go into some of the more lurid ones right now) are the message boards. Websites as varied as Mumsnet and Comparestoreprices.co.uk will carry product reviews of items you're looking to buy – featuring comments and the experiences other new parents have had with these bits and bobs. If you're looking for a baby monitor that will cover a specific range or will work in a room where there's a computer too, or you're just after the opinions of people who've actually used them, instead of the blurb from the shop assistant, then get online and start asking around.

Nursery, Paternity, Upholstery

Pregnancy: Weeks 25–28

At this point your baby will have grown to around 10½ to 12 inches (25–30cm) in length. Your partner will be feeling its kicks and jumps – at first as slight 'fluttering' feelings, then as more vigorous stomps, especially as your baby responds to sounds or to touch. Babies have rapid eye movement (REM) at around 24 weeks – which indicates that they're dreaming. It'll be swallowing some of the amniotic fluid it's encased in and so may get hiccups. Its heartbeat is clearly heard through a stethoscope and you may be able to hear it by putting your ear to your partner's stomach – in the privacy of your own home ideally . . .

Expectancy Explained

The Nursery . . . Or Where Do I Put All This Stuff I've Bought?

The nursery. Cosy, idealistic name applied to the spare room or box room or broom cupboard that's going to be your son or daughter's bedroom for the next few years. The time to prepare the nursery if you've not done it already is **NOW!** That's because from here on in your partner won't be able to shift any furniture for fear of her waters breaking, or else she'll become nauseous at the smell of the paint you're using – while you will also find yourself too on edge before the birth, or knackered afterwards, to plan doing anything more taxing than taking a nap.

HOW SHOULD I DECORATE THE NURSERY?

If you don't know the gender of your baby then you may want to colour the room in a neutral design that you can 'sex up' with murals or pictures after they're born.

You may be tempted to simply plonk the cot in the spare room – beside the exercise bike that's now become a clothes horse – and otherwise leave the 'junk' room as just that, because your baby will only be sleeping in there and won't notice the décor. This is a bad move because:

- **You'll be in here too:** It won't just be your baby who spends time in here. You and your missus will eventually set up camp here to feed, comfort and change your baby. You may sleep in here, off and on, if you're seeking some peace while your partner feeds or settles your wailing offspring, or if you find it wonderfully bonding to watch your kid sleep, though it's most likely you'll just be banished from your own bed for a misdemeanour that's no longer in keeping with your new-found role – so put a comfy chair in there or think twice before relocating the guest bed.

- **It should be a fun room:** Some text books claim that too much stimulation in the nursery will upset your baby's sleep patterns, but by at least making the room a cosy place for your kid to be – a place where they're used to having stories and not a place that you use as a threat – you're more likely to find that they'll go down to sleep a whole lot easier. If you make 'going to bed' a form of punishment you can hardly be surprised that your child won't want to even when they're not in the wrong. Get into the habit of making it a cool room.

- **It should be painted in relaxing shades:** Yellows create a sunny feel even in a dimly lit room but aren't as in your face or overly stimulating as reds or orange colours. Blue also works as a calming colour. If in doubt go with white or cream.

HOW DO I MAKE THE HOUSE 'BABY FRIENDLY'?

The mention of electrical socket covers in the last chapter may sow a seed of nagging doubt about how safe your home is for a new baby. Well, don't panic, there's plenty of time to prepare your home for the stage when your baby's feet make a pitter-patter. But when they are active, they're bursting with months of pent-up action and a sponge of a mind that makes every nook, cranny, plughole and door handle a thing of wonder. At that point you will be back at work toiling to feed that extra mouth and a lot keener on sleeping at weekends than doing DIY. Since you're doing the nursery anyway, you want to add these to your to-do list:

- **Check the temperature:** Position the cot bed away from radiators or direct light from windows – or else turn down the rads and fit a sunshade or blackout blind (£9.99 from www.ikea.com) to the window to stop the room exceeding the recommended temperature. This also makes daytime naps easier. Also, put a fan in here and buy a room thermometer – a Philips Baby Care Digital Bath and Bedroom Thermometer (around £12.50) will also gauge the water temperature for your kid's bath. According to FSID (the Foundation for the Study of Infant Deaths) the room should be kept between 16 and 20°C – so 18°C (65°F) is ideal. Alternatively, the Egg Room Thermometer acts as a night-light and emits warning colours if the temperature gets too hot or cold (£15.50, Boots).

- **Install a carbon monoxide detector:** You should certainly consider investing in a detector, is the advice of Sheila Merrill, Head of Home Safety at the Royal Society for the Prevention of Accidents (www.rospa.com). CO poisoning, which is a silent, invisible and odourless killer, doesn't just result from gas, it can come from any fossil-fuel-burning device, and young children are among the most vulnerable to carbon monoxide poisoning.

- **Fit a smoke alarm:** Ideally a mains-wired system, rather than a battery-operated alarm. Most fire services offer free smoke alarms and installation, and the alarms usually come with long-lasting batteries that are nigh-on impossible to remove.

- **Look out for locks:** As Merrill points out, no safety equipment, no matter how high-tech, is a substitute for supervision. Having said that, items like safety-gates and window locks can go some way in preventing avoidable accidents, particularly involving stairs – it's never too early to prepare and a good start would be to fit locks or safety catches to cupboards storing medicines and bleach.

SHOULD I TRADE IN THE CAR FOR A 'FAMILY' ONE?

The arrival of your new bundle of joy could mean the end of the line for your BMW Z4 sports convertible – to be replaced by something family friendly, more practical and, yes, therefore dull. Motoring journalist Guy Bird has a few key pointers you should bear in mind when tearfully handing over the keys to your soft-top and weighing up which shade to get that Volvo little-people carrier in:

Feel the space

Work out how much room you're going to need – especially boot space if you're going to be carrying a buggy around. According to Bird you should beware of models that favour form over function.

Go for ease of access

For the sake of your spine alone you're better off opting for five-door over three-door models. The back-saving experts also advise parents to sit in the back seat of the car whenever they put their kid in its seat – but they're not the ones who'll be rushing to drop the baby off with Grandma on a Saturday night, so be prepared for some pain and profanities as you get your child in and out of the car. Bird suggests that before you buy your dream machine, try fitting the child-seat then lifting – one-handed – a 10lb bag of potatoes in and out of it half a dozen times just to give you both a feel for things to come.

Think of safety

To see how the car you want to buy will stand up to crashes and side-impacts or to see how much damage it can inflict on a pedestrian, check out the Euro NCAP website www.euroncap. com, which features the safety scores for any make of car according to the European New Car Assessment Programme (not to be mistaken for NCAP, the National Christian Alliance on Prostitution).

Hire one first

Your new-found responsibility as a parent-to-be may lead you to opt for the 'greenest' set of wheels you can find. This may mean you'll pass by the bigger gas guzzlers – but you do so at your peril! Any parent who's gone from a low-seat saloon car to an SUV, Jeep or similar such 'tank' will confirm that it's a whole lot easier for getting kids in and out of.

Check out the upholstery

How easy is it to clean the interior? In the first two and a half years of a child's life they'll produce 250 litres (55 gallons) of urine and an estimated 100kg (220lb) of poo. Admittedly most will stay in the nappy – but some won't. Vomit knows no bounds either. Keep a cloth and cleansing solution in the boot and remember, leather will wipe down more readily than fabric seat covers.

Add an extension

You can get seat-belt extensions for expectant mothers that are in keeping with approved safety standards from suppliers such as www.safetybeltservices.co.uk. Obviously, you're not going to have the time to order one while she's in the throes of another contraction, so make her as comfortable as possible, and phone the hospital if you haven't already to let them know you're on your way.

PATERNITY LEAVE

WHAT IS PATERNITY LEAVE?

According to an Equal Opportunities Commission (EOC) survey 23 per cent of men don't realise that they're entitled to time off when their baby is born.

In short, it's the fortnight that fathers take off after their child is born. Depending on the kind of dad you are it's treated either as: (a) a crucial time in which you can support your partner in her recovery from the trauma of labour and childbirth and for you to form a bond with your baby or (b) handy for catching up with DIY and a few DVD box sets.

At the moment the law allows you to take up to two weeks off work as 'paid' paternity leave. However, you should read the small print on this one. To qualify:

- You must be the biological father – or at least the mother's husband/legal partner.

- You are going to be responsible for the child and you're taking time off to care for the child or support the mother (even if you do end up tiling the bathroom for two weeks).

- You must be an employee and have worked for the firm for 26 weeks by the end of the 15th week before the baby is due. (To find the 15th week before the baby is due look in a diary for the Sunday before your child's EDD then start counting back 15 weeks – that'll be the start of the 15th week.)

What paternity pay do I get?

Not a lot. Employed fathers who tick all the boxes above are entitled to Statutory Paternity Pay (SPP) of £139.58, or 90% of their average weekly earnings (whichever is lower) as of 2016 – for two weeks only. Barely enough to cover the nappies in the first week. The same EOC survey found that 41 per cent of new dads couldn't afford to take time off after the birth. Some employers top up this payment – though they get refunded only the SPP amount by HM Revenue and Customs. Others can make life quite difficult for men seeking paternity leave – one in five employees claim this has been the case when they've asked for time off even though, by law, most working fathers are entitled to it. Many dads will opt for taking some of their annual leave around the time the baby is born in a bid not to lose out on vital funds.

The UK allowance for dads to have time off is generous compared to some nations – in the USA, for example, there's no such state-backed system – but in Sweden fathers can take up to eight months off work to share in their child's upbringing. The Swedish scheme encourages firms to pay extended leave on top of the government payments and is partly designed to enable working women to return to their jobs sooner.

What if I'm self-employed?

While most employees are entitled to paternity leave and many family-friendly firms encourage dads to take more time off or work more flexible hours, there's no state-funded leave allowance for self-employed dads. Some freelance fathers-to-be adjust their budgets in the months leading up to the birth in order to cover them for time out when the baby's born. You should also investigate what you're entitled to in the way of benefits and tax credits too (see Chapter 8 for a full list of ways to ease the cost of having a baby).

When do I tell the boss I'm taking my leave?

Officially you need to tell the firm that you're taking paternity leave by the end of the 15th week before the baby is due. To get the Statutory Paternity Pay (SPP) you need to give your boss 28 days' notice as well as notice in writing stating:

- When the baby is due
- Whether you're taking one week or two off
- When you want the leave to start

To apply for leave and SPP there's a form available from the www.gov.uk website entitled Ordinary Statutory Paternity Pay and Leave: becoming a birth parent (SC3).

HOW DO I BALANCE WORK WITH THE PREGNANCY?

If you're an expectant dad working full-time the chances are you'll be attending at least one (most likely more) of the following events:

- Midwife appointments
- Scans – 12-week and 20-week at least
- Antenatal classes
- The birth
- Paternity leave
- Registering the birth
- Inoculations post-birth
- Ad hoc appointments in the case of complications or concerns

Since most of these take place during the working day – except the antenatal classes you attend with your partner – you may have to fine-tune a juggling act here. Begin by letting your boss know that you're about to become a dad as soon as you can. Also inform your line manager and Human Resources department – partly as an administrative formality and also to see what specific rights or perks your firm may offer prospective dads. According to Jo Lyon, a maternity and paternity leave advisor for executive firm Talking Talent, it may be better for you to talk to your HR department first – to elicit their views and support – and get advice on any procedure for delivering the news to your boss. It all sounds a little threatening but the truth is most modern firms are pretty accommodating to the demands put upon new dads – after all, many bosses are parents, most are even human. In fact it's often the expectant dads themselves, hard-wired to stay in the office for long hours at all costs, who deprive themselves of time to share in a few magical moments along the pregnancy path.

It's understandable. The pressure to keep a hold on your job has probably never been greater – with an extra mouth to feed, clothe, fit out with a nursery and provide wheels for. Your partner could be giving up work or at least likely to have a dip in her income and, no matter how much you want to be involved in the pregnancy, you're going to have to deal with more demands on the work, home and finance front.

To decide how you're going to balance work and the womb be sure to sit down with your partner and decide which appointments you think are most important to attend. Remember also that the hospital and the midwives or doctors call the shots on the timing of these things – it can be difficult to rearrange sessions at short notice, especially if your partner is working too, so be prepared for missing out on some key checkups or even scans.

Get your workmates on board

Make them aware of the fact that you're taking time out to help with the pregnancy or attend things like scans. Enlist their support to ensure that you have cover when you go to events – and be sure to invite them to the 'head-wetting' as a way of saying thanks.

Talk to colleagues who've been there

Ask them how they did it and what worked for them when it came to balancing work and home life. They may also know of any perks your company provides for parents such as flexitime arrangements.

Get things in perspective

In this economic climate, taking time off can feel more difficult and can make some people feel more vulnerable at work. But, as Jo Lyon points out, having a baby for the first time is a one-off experience that you can never have again, so you really need to make the most of it. What it might mean is that you go only to appointments you feel are crucial and that you work around the business requirements to an extent to take your paternity leave, but it should not mean that you don't feel able to take reasonable time off.

What if the baby arrives late or early?

The sight of you suddenly dashing from your desk, mid-morning, with a look of horrified panic and mumbling about 'not even bought the cot yet' should give your work-mates a hint that the birth date has come forward unexpectedly. This is likely to be a source of great amusement to them.

But you're also officially obliged to tell the big cheese if your baby has been born prematurely. Informing your HR department or line manager about this during a sudden dash to the hospital won't be at the forefront of your mind. But when it's 'reasonably practical', as the government literature puts it, you should let them know if you're commencing your paternity leave from that point and not planning on returning to work for a week or two.

Equally, you must give notice as soon as possible if your baby hasn't arrived and you need to shift your paternity leave dates. Pregnancies are full of false alarms so you may find yourself tearing off to the hospital, only to return to work the next day cursing whoever Braxton Hicks was and his confounded contractions. Again, keep your employer and any colleagues who'll be covering you in the loop. Should you encounter any problems speak to your company's HR department . . . if it has one.

Your paternity leave must finish within 56 days of the birth.

WHAT IS SHARED PARENTAL LEAVE?

Since April 2015, couples have been able to divide almost all the traditional maternity leave entitlement between them as Shared Parental Leave (SPL). Aside from the compulsory fortnight recovery period new mothers must take after childbirth, the remaining 50 can be divvied up between parents in any combination. A maximum of 37 weeks is covered by Shared Parental Pay (ShPP) and you can take time off together or separately. But one year on from its introduction just 1% of eligible dads had taken up SPL, citing such reasons as it being 'financially unworkable ' or 'mothers refusing to share their maternity leave.' Confusion over ShPP – despite a calculator on the GOV website – haven't helped. Many hold the opinion that, in reality, the SPL is inferior to other European versions. (Scottish football fans have said so for years.) If you fancy it see www.working-families.org.uk

TRAVEL

CAN WE STILL FLY WHEN SHE'S PREGNANT?

If you've got a holiday overseas booked or you're hoping to surprise her with a short break that involves somebody else's air space then there are a few things you should definitely know.

First off, jabs. Your partner may well be sick of the sight of needles by now after the various tests and checkups she'll have been through. So she may not take kindly to having to endure a long list of inoculations in order for her to combat a host of exotic diseases – more importantly, she may not be able to have any jabs. The Royal College of Obstetricians and Gynaecologists have outlined the vaccines that pregnant women can have along with some vaccines, which are usually live, that aren't safe for her – including polio (oral), typhoid (oral), yellow fever and MMR – that could harm the baby.

If you're going to fly then now – the second trimester – is the time to do it, according to the Royal College of Midwives (RCM), which has advised airlines such as British Airways on the issue of pregnancy and flying. Many airlines do accept pregnant women but have a cut-off point, which is usually after 34 weeks. However, you or your partner need to check with your chosen airline direct and ask them at what point she would not be allowed to fly. (It could be anything from 25 weeks up to 35 – it depends on the airline.) Because of the possibility of some women going into premature labour when they fly, either due to the change in the air composition in the aircraft or high altitude, the RCM maintain that it's impossible to say for definite whether an individual mother should fly at a specific time.

Whether you decide to fly or not, if you're travelling overseas when she's pregnant take care to check your travel insurance details if you're going abroad while she's expecting. If you're stranded in mainland Europe because your partner is giving birth to your baby there may be hospital costs for you to pay – especially if it's born premature and requires specialist treatment. Find out which countries have reciprocal health arrangements that cover births or else check out what insurance you can get to cover the costs of your baby being born in foreign climes.

IF WE CAN'T JET OFF FOR A WEEKEND BREAK, HOW ELSE CAN I TREAT HER?

Aside from doing the vacuuming and back rubs? You could look into a short break that doesn't involve flying, perhaps to a hotel offering pampering services for pregnant women. Websites such as www.babycentre.co.uk list hotels and spas that provide specialist massages and treatments designed to deal with fluid retention, fatigue, stretch marks and a whole load of other stuff you really don't want to know about.

7

Tales of the Unexpected

Pregnancy: Weeks 29-32

At this point your baby will measure 13 to 16 inches (33–40cm) in length from head to bum and weigh around 3lb (1.4kg). Its eyelids will open for the first time around this stage. You can't see them, of course, but light-skinned babies will have blue eyes and dark-skinned ones are more likely to be brown. Its head hair will be starting to grow – just as its father is tearing out the last of his. A baby is well within the 'viable' stage at this time – meaning that if it were born now it would have a good chance of survival. By now the connection between the part of your baby's brain that's responsible for emotion and the thinking part (the cerebral cortex) is established. Much to your partner's delight, it can now roll over in the womb . . .

Expectancy Explained

Braxton Hicks Contractions

It's the final trimester and, although unlikely, your baby could appear at any time – but the 'Braxton Hicks' contractions that pregnant women experience at this time are false ones. They're named after the doctor who identified them in 1872 and are designed to prepare the mother's body for the forthcoming 'Big Push'. Because your baby is growing very rapidly now your partner will be feeling increasingly tired – and since the baby will cause her discomfort at night, she'll be losing out on much-needed sleep too. She may also experience bleeding gums, heartburn, flatulence, indigestion, increased clumsiness, a protruding navel and piles. It's at about this point that you may start hatching your 'escape plan'. But now is the time when the expectant dad comes into his own, when he can step up to the plate and reveal himself to be a wise and capable dad-to-be among his peers . . . because now is the time for the antenatal classes!

DO I REALLY NEED TO GO TO ANTENATAL CLASSES?

Depending on how you look at it, it's either the perfect opportunity to find out all you need to know about birth and beyond in one hit (aside from reading this book) while also making friends with similarly terrified parents-to-be, or a complete waste of time in which a domineering midwife contradicts all you've read so far while forcing a doll's head through a plastic cervix.

Despite having a reputation for being something like a pre-labour love-in, where expectant dads simply turn up to show willing, these sessions do have their uses. You'll learn what to do for her in the early throes of labour, when to come into hospital and what to expect – you'll also get a heads-up on some of the common problems that occur during birth and the different types of delivery.

Did you know?

Get to Class!

Fathers attending antenatal classes are shown to be more knowledgeable and better prepared for the birth and decisions about baby feeding choices according to a study by Fathers Direct.

If I can only attend one class, which should it be?

Midwives generally agree that the answer to this is the one with 'the labour talk'. Ask the midwife or class co-ordinator at which point she (or he) will be covering this topic and be sure to get along.

This will be the most demanding part for the father – prepare to wince a lot – and this class will also cover postnatal stuff. According to Melvyn Dunstall the most commonly asked question from fathers-to-be at classes is 'When can we have sex again?' Midwives will discuss this as it also gives them an opportunity to cover methods of contraception – it's useful to remind yourself of this too, because your partner will be able to conceive another baby almost immediately after her pregnancy.

If nothing else, be sure to take away the following from an antenatal class:

- Some biscuits.
- Answers to any questions that have come up during the last few months – or to your current anxieties about the birth. Even ones of a sensitive nature can be covered by the midwife if you ask for a one-to-one chat at the end.
- Phone numbers or email addresses of other expectant dads in the class. No matter what 'type' of expectant dad they

are – Mr Know-all-the-answers, Mr Phantom-pregnancy, Mr Could-not-give-a-toss, you'll have your own ideas about the couples around you – antenatal-group friendships can actually prove useful. You may well find that you and another dad from the group end up trading surplus baby items, babysitting each other's kids or sharing a sympathetic pint or two.

- Something out of it. There are plenty of dads who'll tell you how these classes were a waste of time or how the midwife spoke only to their partner. But if you see these groups for their real worth to you – as a talking shop to fill in the knowledge gaps you and your partner have – then they can be a real bonus.

Do I need to do a tour of the labour ward?

If the antenatal class is taking place at the hospital where your partner's having the baby you may be offered a tour of the maternity facilities. If she's having a water birth there you'll be shown the birthing pool too – so long as it's not in use at the time. Remember, there's always a chance you won't be there to take your partner to hospital if she goes into labour – you may have to give directions to someone else, over the phone. Get a SatNav-like familiarity with the location.

- Ask about where the family waiting area is, in case your in-laws tag along.
- Find out about car parking. Does the hospital operate a pass system? If not, what are parking charges?
- Check out where the vending machines are. Labour can seem to last longer than an entire Netflix series at times. Both your partner and you will need some sustenance, so make a note of where the snack bars are.

Are all classes the same?

Each antenatal group will differ in some way. Usually the personality and preferences of the health professional who's running it will have some influence on things. The National Childbirth Trust – with around 380 branches in the UK – is one of the most commonly available but it's not free. Prices vary according to where you live and which of the range of courses on offer you go for – but a basic first-time-parents course for both of you will cost from around £129 per pair for 16 to 20 hours of tuition. Other private-practice courses include Daddy Natal antenatal classes for men, aquanatal, yoga-based classes and even 'Hypno-birthing' groups where you're taught to use hypnosis to ease her pain. Contact the ones you like the sound of and ask for a breakdown of what they cover and when the classes take place. Also ask your partner to speak to the midwife, as there are likely to be some FREE classes on offer at the hospital. The hospital classes will in most cases offer a 'tour' of the labour ward or 'birthing suite' or whatever term your hospital uses for the screaming zone. Parents not attending hospital antenatal classes can arrange a tour by contacting the hospital direct.

When do these classes take place?

They usually start running at the end of the second trimester (27th week) but you need to book a place on them a lot earlier to get a time slot that suits you. Most take place after work – though some are available during the day or at weekends – and are taught by midwives, health visitors, nurses or specialist antenatal 'coaches'.

EXPECTANT DADS' EXPERIENCES

Men-only Classes

Aside from the Daddy Natal groups the NCT and a number of regional health groups have devised one-off classes just for fathers-to-be to attend. These are usually called 'Partners Sessions' since they're aimed at birthing partners – not necessarily fathers-to-be. Don't be surprised if you turn up and the mother, 'bezzie mate' or lodger of a local lass who's due the same time as your partner is there too. Here five fathers-to-be explain what happens during them:

'I feared it would be like a therapy session for the dads-to-be, but it was much more practical than that. We were shown (with the aid of various props and pictures) what had been going on inside our women's insides and what would happen (hopefully) during a natural birth. It explained a lot of the reasons for the aches and pains that Mel had told me about at various stages through the birth.'

Matthew D

'I liked the fact that this was our first meeting and that we had yet to meet as couples, so we've met each other as "blokes" rather than the partner of a pregnant woman – it made a difference to how we reacted to each other. I felt that I was more able to speak about things that had been going through my mind with regard to the pregnancy than I would if I'd just been down the pub with a bunch of mates. I was surprised at how open everyone was, to be honest. It helps that we didn't have any preconceptions of each other and that we only had a short time. It focused the mind and made it easier to speak openly.'

Paul S

'I was really surprised how everyone had relatively similar concerns. I'm a bit squeamish and it helped that within a couple of minutes half of the others had mentioned that they were too. It helped to give me the confidence that I am not too different from others and will be fine. After the first few minutes the discussion was flowing and everyone was very open and had a good laugh along the way. As we were having a home birth the NCT organiser suggested that I watch a home birth on YouTube. I watched several in the end and they didn't make me pass out. In fact, the extra knowledge that I gained from this meant that there were no surprises when the baby came. I was able to be calm and understood what was happening at each stage. I didn't feel faint.'

Charley G

'Friends I had spoken to said "Do the class, it is really good." I thought it might be too new-age for me, but found the instructor, information, pictures, explanations, a chance to look at needles and other equipment reassuring – it helps to know what happens in detail to reduce surprise and stress on the day. It was good to have other blokes in the room as well. Some things shared go to show that you are not alone with any pregnancy quirks you or your partner might have.'

Tom L

'The key points that were useful to me were: the timing of the contractions (i.e. when you should go to the hospital), the fact that the delivery room will be very hot (so wear appropriate clothing), that you can get a pass for the car park at the hospital and the breathing stuff during labour.'

Dominic N

WHERE DO I FIGURE IN THE BIRTH PLAN?

Part of the class will cover the 'birth plan'. Birth plans are useful in enabling women to put down their needs, wants and wishes in advance. Your partner may consider them as gospel. Unfortunately, not everyone at the hospital will – that's where you come in.

Labour can last for hours – in some cases, technically days (yep, plural). During this time there'll be several changes in shift among the hospital staff. The chances are the midwife you first see when you arrive at the hospital won't be the same one your baby first sees when it arrives in the world.

As a result you're going to be one of the few consistent things for your partner during the labour – which is why you need to know what her wishes are when it comes to her master plan. Melvyn Dunstall suggests your partner goes through her plan with the midwife before she goes into labour to discuss what her best options are.

Your role during the actual birth will be on a par with the trainer of a boxer at ring-side – you're there to mop her brow and offer words of support, but you can't really do any of the punching – or pushing in this case – yourself. However, you can do your bit to ensure her wishes are met by constantly communicating with the midwife.

Make a note – either mental or written – to check that what your partner wants to happen when she's in labour does happen, especially when she's too agonised to ask herself. Find out the following now:

- What pain medication does she want to have? (Find out what the hospital offers too. Some may not offer epidurals – a super-painkiller administered by an anaesthetist – if they've not been booked in advance.)
- Would she like to have anyone else at the hospital? This may not always be possible, but even you as the

father-to-be will need to take a break for a moment or two during a long labour, so if there's anyone else nearby who can support her make a note of their phone number.

- What position would she most like to be in to have the baby?
- Does she want to hold the baby the moment it's born?
- Does she mind if students are present at the birth? (Medical ones, not just any old nosy undergraduate oik.)
- What are her opinions on having a caesarean? An episiotomy? A forceps or ventouse delivery?
- Does she want you – yes, you, Expectant Dad – to cut the umbilical cord?
- How would she like to give your baby its first feed? Breast or bottle?

If nothing else reading this should make you flip to the 'Glossary' section to find out what the 'ventouse' involves. While you can make a note of these things, and on the whole most of her wishes will be met, be prepared to compromise a little during the birth. Labour and birth are always unpredictable and midwife Melvyn is among those who believe there is nothing worse than a husband saying, 'She does not want an epidural,' when the reality of his partner's pain exceeds what they were expecting. When it comes to the birth plan go with the flow – don't be afraid to ask questions, but listen to the midwife. And don't be at all surprised if it's your partner who ditches the plan once things start hotting up.

SHOULD I FILM MY CHILD BEING BORN?

This topic has led to combat scenes on the labour ward in the past when medical teams competed with budding Steven Spielbergs to get a first glimpse of the head. In the end, it's got to be your partner's call as to whether you actually film the birth of your baby or just take a snapshot of mother and baby's first moments that she can 'touch up' in Photoshop later. If you are taking a camera along or using a camera phone to capture the magic moment remember to:

- **Pack it:** Put 'camera phone!' on the list of things for the overnight bag (see Chapter 8) and pack it!
- **Charge it:** Or have batteries to hand for a camera – the hospital won't take kindly to you unplugging the incubator so you can juice up your phone.
- **Check it's OK:** The medical staff may object to you wielding a camera around the room, especially if you're using a flash – get the OK first. Don't even bother taking the sound boom.
- **Be patient:** Allow your partner some time to compose herself – hair and make-up – if she wants to before you take any pictures. There should ideally be a mirror in the 'overnight bag' too – though that's not the reason why it's there . . . all will be revealed on that one.

WHAT'S BEST, HOME OR HOSPITAL BIRTH?

Your partner will ask you this if she's in two minds about it. She'll possibly have decided anyway and be asking you out of nothing more than common courtesy. More worrying is that she may be asking for your genuine, long-pondered thoughts on this matter! So here's a bluffer's guide on the topic.

Often the father's opinion will carry a fair bit of weight in this matter – especially if he's worried about his partner's well-being at home.

While the final say will usually be with the mother, Professor Patrick O'Brien says he's seen many women who were keen on a home birth decide against it just because they could see the father was terrified by the prospect.

There are a number of factors for you and your partner to discuss-cum-have a blazing row over when it comes to turning your home into a maternity ward.

- **Is your home adequate?** You've got to ask yourselves where the birth will take place. Is the room big enough? Is it easy to keep warm? How do you minimise the mess from waters breaking or blood loss?

- **Water birth:** If you're planning a home 'water birth' you need to check to see if the structure of the house is strong enough to support a large amount of water. Plus you need to consider how you are going to fill it and keep the water at the right temperature. And then empty it.

- **It's great if she hates hospitals:** Your partner gets to have the baby in a comfortable, familiar environment, which should relax her (and therefore you too) a little more.

- **Refreshments:** You'll need lots of tea and biscuits because your partner and baby will – ideally – be attended by two midwives for a home birth.

- **There's less panic:** You don't have to make a decision about when to go to hospital or risk having her going into labour during a hellish trek stuck in traffic while she swears and tears the upholstery in the back.

- **There are no drugs:** Well, not the real 'class A' painkillers at least. There's very little likelihood of the baby being delivered using pain-relieving drugs – and certainly not by Caesarean – if it's born at home. This point is the key one to chew over. While many first-time mothers say they don't want to have pain relief before the birth, plenty of them opt for it when it's offered later in the labour. This won't be an option if she's having the baby at home. One study into home birth, by the National Birthday Trust Fund, found that about 40 per cent of first-time mothers needed to transfer from home to hospital.

- **It's a growing trend:** The most recent ONS data for

England and Wales for 2007 report that home births have risen among mums under 30 since 2004 – the NHS is pushing, for want of a better phrase, for more women to give birth at home.

- **It's safe:** Home deliveries are – statistically – as safe as hospital deliveries for women with uncomplicated pregnancies where the GP or midwife doesn't envisage any complications. Research from the Netherlands and NHS data shows that there was no difference in the death rates of either mothers or babies in over half a million births studied.

- **It's still quite rare though:** Despite the rise, only 2.3 per cent of the 695,233 live births in England and Wales in 2014 were home ones.

Did you know?

Water Way to Arrive

There is no danger of your baby drowning during a water birth as it only takes its first breath when it encounters air that's different in temperature from its body.

Did you know?

They Don't Smack Babies

Whether it's at hospital or home one of the first things that will happen when your baby is born is that the midwife will give it a rub with a towel to change its temperature and so trigger the breathing mechanism. Any thoughts you had of seeing your kid dangled upside down and smacked in order to get it crying and so open up its lungs are now dashed.

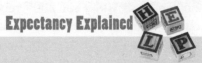

Expectancy Explained

Prepare to Deal with the Public . . .

The conception of a child is a very intimate thing, of course. Birth, despite the crowd, is something uniquely special to you and your child's mother too. But the bit in between, the pregnancy, is a matter for open public debate, it seems. Once you're a pregnant pairing you can kiss goodbye to your own privacy laws. You suddenly become public property and get a slight glimpse of what it must be like to be a paparazzi-poked celebrity.

The most common example of this is the hands-on approach people, and by this I mean complete strangers, suddenly have towards your partner's bump. At this stage of the pregnancy it becomes an unnervingly common event. The bigger your partner's bump, the more people seem to home in on it. It's as if, like the girl in the film *Children of Men*, she's the last expectant woman on earth. Loosely connected friends, distant relatives and especially old women at bus stops will start spontaneous inquisitions. They'll begin with blunt questions about stuff that the pair of you may not even have discussed yourselves such as your baby's sex, possible names, type of birth, type of contraception that failed you so dramatically etc. Some will tell you what the sex of your child will be – without you even asking – based solely on mystic 'old wives' guesswork that revolves around how low or high the foetus is lying. Finally, all – without fail and certainly without consideration towards your partner's feelings or yours – will reach out and rub the bump.

HOW DO I GIVE THE PERFECT BACK RUB?

Back rubs. Not something you'll necessarily get a crash course in at the antenatal class, but a vital skill in the armoury of the expectant dad all the same. The pressure of her ever enlarging uterus – coupled with the increasing weight of your child – can play havoc with your partner's back and leg muscles around this time.

This in turn leads to a strain on her sciatic nerve, followed by sharp pains around her lower back and buttocks and a further drop in her tolerance threshold when it comes to you. To win back some Brownie points, supply a little hands-on therapy:

- Have her sit on a stool with a cushion or, if you have one, a fitness ball (also called a Swiss ball).

- Take your place behind her, on the sofa or a chair, placing your hands at the base of her spine while looking over her shoulder at the match on the TV.

- If she's not going to play ball with that one then have her lie down on the bed, on her side, with a pillow supporting her bump.

- Then work your way up one side of her back using gentle rubs up to and across her shoulders. According to Alissia Harvey, massage specialist at The Elms spa near Worcester, which runs specialist soon-to-be-parent pampering sessions, your partner can get pregnancy-friendly massage oils for just this purpose.

- Expectant fathers should avoid being too heavy-handed when providing a little relief in this way. Harvey suggests you gently use the 'heel' of your hand or your knuckles but keep it very soft, don't try to penetrate like a sports massage.

- Harvey suggests a massaging man doesn't neglect his partner's buttocks or thighs (like we would?). Again, take time to perform slow, sweeping, light-pressure rubs around these aching points for her.

- Listen out for the 'Ooo, there! That's it.' Then execute a few targeted rubs and kneading using your thumbs, working in small, deep circles.

Be aware that you may find yourself asked to do foot rubs too. Not half as much fun, but one way of cutting the amount of time you have to do this for her is to have her wrap her feet in a damp flannel or cloth or a bowl of warm soapy water. This reduces the swelling and eases some of the soreness.

Let your fingers do the working

Among some of the many humorous anecdotes of 'how we killed time during pregnancy' you may or may not wish to share with friends is how you helped with her perineal massage. This helps her prepare for childbirth and may reduce the risk of her needing an episiotomy. Expectant mothers and their partners will try massaging her perineum (the area between the vagina and rectum). This isn't something midwives recommend as such since there's no scientifically proven benefit to it – though that's not stopped many couples from giving it a try. It's helpful – but not compulsory.

EXPECTANT DADS' EXPERIENCES

Getting the Feel for Fatherhood

'I do feel part of the pregnancy, Mel has been really good at telling me everything that's going on and every time the baby moves when we're at home together she shows me or grabs my hand so I can feel it too. In the early days when she got little "pops" in her belly Mel worked out a way to share it with me – it may sound a little strange but it worked. She'd tap the inside of my cheek with her finger lightly, to give me an idea of the feeling. I have been to all of the midwife and doctor meetings. I was with Mel, walking

her to work, when she had her first Braxton Hicks. I have taken over all of the household chores – cooking, cleaning, washing etc. – and generally made sure that Mel has what she needs when she needs it. I've tried not to be too overbearing when we're out and about, but haven't always succeeded in that!' Matthew D

WHAT SHALL WE CALL OUR BABY?

Whole books have been written on this subject alone. Not exactly gripping page-turners, admittedly, but they highlight how important a subject it is to us all. There are no rules as such to choosing the name for your child. A wander around any play-ground these days will confirm that kids' names can be influenced by fashion, nostalgia, reality TV and what in some cases seems like out-and-out cruelty. The question: 'Thought of any names yet?' will come your way soon after: 'What are you having, a boy or a girl?' Of course, the answer to the latter will usually deter-mine the former – but if you don't know the sex of your baby yet there's still plenty of fun to be had sitting down with your part-ner and a book of baby names and seeing which ones provoke a kick or womb-stretching cartwheel from your kid.

A few things for you to consider include:

- **How does it 'scan'?** Try saying, out loud, some of the first names you have in mind with your surname – or whatever surname your baby will have. If you're not married yet, but could be in the future, then take into account how your child's name will sound if you're going to change it or double-barrel it.

- **Test it for nicknames.** Think about how your child's name could be shortened to a nickname too – and see the names below found following a trawl of phone records. Take them as a warning.

- **Any family heirlooms to add?** Maintaining a family trad-ition is often a reason why so-called 'older' names make a reappearance. Relatives may drop heavy hints, but don't be pressured into naming your child after them – unless you know it could influence your place in their will.

- **Do the 'telling off' test.** No matter how well behaved you think your child will be as they grow up you are still going to have to shout out their name, in public, every time you need to stop them doing something dangerous, spiteful or some distance away. Rehearse shouting out your child's name (as a dad it will be your duty to shout anyway) and see how comfortable you feel with it. Suddenly 'Lavender Boo' or 'Princess Apricot' – or whatever latest trendy name all the celebs are using for their kids – won't seem so attractive.

What were you thinking of?

Genuine unfortunate names, discovered by TheBabyWebsite.com:

Justin Case	Anna Sasin	Tim Burr
Terry Bull	Rose Bush	Barb Dwyer
Paige Turner	Carrie Oakey	Stan Still
Mary Christmas	Priti Manek	

What if we're struggling to agree on names?

Your partner may be set on a name that you don't like, or vice versa. One way of airing your concerns about a name is suggesting that you and she write out lists of your favourites for boys and girls. Swap your lists and cross out the ones you don't like, then use the ones left to create a 'shortlist'. You don't have to name your baby at the birth so don't sweat it if you can't decide as yet. Quite often even having a name in mind before the birth doesn't guarantee that it'll stick once your child is born. Finally clamping eyes on your baby for the first time – realising the similarities they may share with one of you or just the look of their 'character' – can be enough for you to rethink calling him Colin.

HOW DO I KNOW IF I'M SUFFERING FROM A 'PHANTOM PREGNANCY'?

It's a term you'll hear bandied about a lot right now, in particular when you have the audacity to complain about the odd ache or twinge you've been having. She'll pass a comment about you suffering from a phantom or sympathetic pregnancy. Though she'll probably put the emphasis on the 'pathetic'.

But there's plenty of research to suggest that at least one in 10 expectant dads do suffer from some form of 'couvade syndrome' – taken from the French word for hatching – in which they mirror their partner's symptoms.

Studies carried out on 282 expectant fathers at St George's University in London revealed that those men 'suffering' from phantom pregnancies reported experiencing back pains, nausea and sickness, cravings, weight gain and even false contractions!

The good news is that these feelings pass as the pregnancy progresses (so you won't need to book a double birthing pool) and are, according to some psychologists, simply a subconscious way of getting you focused on the whole pregnancy process that has become slightly overcooked.

Phantom pregnancy can be understood as an extreme form of empathy, according to psychologist Russell Hurn. He maintains that it occurs when the expectant father literally experiences the pain of their partner as physical sensations have been re-created by his mind after receiving emotional material from the mother-to-be. In Hurn's view affected men are essentially reading their partner at a deep and unconscious level and their body then re-creates the information. Sadly this explanation won't wash with her when you nick her pregnancy pillow for the umpteenth time.

8 The Final Countdown

Pregnancy: Weeks 33-36

By this point your baby should have eased up on the somersaults and will be lying – head down – in your partner's womb. He or she may have 'engaged' (dropped down into your partner's pelvis area) ready for birth. Your baby should weigh around 5½lb (2.5kg) – it's gaining weight at a rate of around half an ounce (15g) a day now – and will measure about 21 inches (53cm). By the 36th week it'll have become quite sensitive to light and noise from outside the womb. Most are probably itching to get out – certainly your partner will start using phrases like 'fed up' and 'want to get it over with' a lot more.

If your baby hasn't appeared yet then it's pretty imminent. (If it has then hopefully you'll have skipped through to Chapter 9 and proved yourself to be a wised-up and invaluable birthing partner thanks to everything you read there.) The final few weeks will be spent stocking up on essential supplies for the forthcoming months (SKY+ subscription, DVDs, home-brewing kit etc.), making final touches so your home is baby ready and possibly answering quick-fire questions from your partner-turned-Alan-Sugar-interrogator about your role in the birth plan! In between all this it'll pay for you both to check out any entitlements you should be signed up for in order for you to pay for all this.

HOW WILL WE AFFORD THIS BABY?

There are a number of financial support services on offer to new parents in the UK. These are paid to working parents as well as those who are unemployed or unable to work. Working out how much you should get and how to get it can be a task that makes having the baby look like a walk in the park by comparison, but even if you don't think you qualify for any additional income you should check on your rights regarding the following:

Child Tax Credits (CTC)

You may be entitled to a get a basic amount of £545 a year, which incidentally is the amount new parents can expect to spend on disposable nappies in the first 12 months. You could get extra elements on top of this but how much you get depends on things like your income and circumstances up to £2,780 – you're not eligible if you're claiming Universal Credit though.

Working Tax Credits (WTC)

You could get Working Tax Credits if you're aged from 16 to 24 and have a child – but you must work a certain number of hours a week, get paid for the work you do (or expect to) and have an income below a certain level.

Once again there's an online calculator parents can use at the Gov.UK website, though the process of claiming is still considered by many to be a demoralising experience designed to put people off doing it. But for those in need at this particular time of life-change it's worth the aggro as the potential additional income – the basic amount of Working Tax Credits is up to £1,960 a year – will come in very handy. Some self-employed workers can claim WTCs and with this allowance you could get more (or less) depending on your circumstances and income – though if you're claiming Universal Credit already you won't be eligible for WTCs. Whatever your circumstance do look online or call the Tax Credits office to clarify your chances of receiving these.

Child Benefit

This is paid for every child – the eldest or only child receives £20.70 a week and any additional children get £13.70 each (as of 2016). It's tax-free – but parents with an individual income exceeding £50k (not their combined wages) may pay a charge. It's paid monthly until the child reaches 16 and can be claimed once you've registered your child's birth.

What's a Junior ISA?

The Junior ISA is a tax-free account parents can use in order to save money for their children to have when they're older. They were originally established to replace the Child Trust Fund (CTFs) when parents would receive a one-off payment voucher – to the value of £250 – to set up a trust fund for their newborn baby. The £250 savings incentive and the CTFs have been abolished – in their place are two types of Junior ISA:

- a cash Junior ISA, ie you won't pay tax on interest on the cash you save
- a stocks and shares Junior ISA, ie your cash is invested and you won't pay tax on any capital growth or dividends you receive

Your child can have one or both types of Junior ISA and parents or guardians with parental responsibility can open a Junior ISA and manage the account, but the money belongs to the child. Your child can take control of the account when they're 16, but can't withdraw the money until they turn 18.

Because family and friends may want to give money as a gift to your child on birthdays etc a Junior ISA can be quite a useful piggy bank for parents. Anyone can pay money into a Junior ISA – but the total amount paid in can't go over £4,080. (As of the 2016–17 tax year). So if a benevolent grandparent pays £1,000 into your junior's Junior ISA, only a further £3,080 could be paid into either their cash or stocks and shares Junior ISA in the same tax year.

WHAT ELSE IS MY PARTNER ENTITLED TO?

All women are entitled to free prescriptions and free NHS dental care during pregnancy and for 12 months after the birth of their baby. (In Scotland, Wales and Northern Ireland it's free prescriptions at all times). She'll need to complete a Maternity Exemption form (FW8) – available from the doctor or midwife – to get this.

New mums are entitled to Statutory Maternity Pay (SMP) for a total of 39 weeks out of the 52 weeks of Statutory Maternity Leave. SMP provides 90 per cent of her average weekly earnings (before tax) for the first six weeks followed by £139.58 or 90% of her average weekly earnings (whichever is lower) for the next 33 weeks. Her employer may offer more than SMP – she'll need to discuss this with her firm's HR department before she takes her leave.

Be prepared for your partner to be doubly anxious at this time if she's leaving work to go on maternity leave. Aside from the change of routine and day-to-day interaction she may also be wondering if she will have a job to go back to. A 2015 report by the Equality and Human Rights Commission says around 54,000 new mums lose their jobs across Britain every year. For more information on her entitlements visit www.gov.uk/working-when-pregnant-your-rights

Did you know?

At a Glance: The Cost of a Baby

Several surveys – including ones by AXA Bank and American Express – put the cost of a new baby in its first year between £2,500 and £5,000. Here's where the money goes:

Pregnancy clothes and toiletries	£177
Nursery furniture, decorating, cot and bedding	£410
Buggy	£233
Car seat	£79
Nappies	£500
Baby skin-care products	£380
Formula milk	£600
Food	£360
Baby clothes	£280
Total:	£3,019

EXPECTANT DADS' EXPERIENCES

Making Adjustments

'Nothing is particularly tough – so far – for me at least. But some things have needed a lot of patience and adjustment: tiredness in the first and now third trimesters, economising and saving ready for going down to one salary, and having a lot less sex.'   Charley G

Expectancy Explained

The Nesting Instinct

Cleaning or obsessive-compulsive dusting disorder will become the order of the day for the final couple of months as your partner starts 'nesting'. Along with cravings and morning sickness, nesting is again something that affects some women more than others. The act itself is, as its name suggests, simply cleaning and making the final preparations to your home for your new arrival. However, since your partner is now waddling around like a Jersey dairy cow with trapped wind, she's going to enlist you into many of the more arduous tasks.

Set aside time at the weekends or in the evenings to help out with chores and in particular give yourself plenty of time to put together the nursery furniture. Anecdotal evidence among new fathers shows that flat-pack cots or 'easy assembly' changing tables can take anything from an hour to an entire weekend to put together. Be prepared to sacrifice a few golf mornings in the build-up to the birth too.

WHY DO I NEED A LIST FOR HER OVERNIGHT BAG?

Fold the corner of this page or place a bookmark at this point. What follows is a list of the essential mother and new baby items that your partner will need if she's going to have a hospital birth. In the ideal birth scenario she'll have her overnight hospital bag packed and ready to go once the balloon goes up.

(Some keen mums-to-be start packing this within about a week of conception.) If not then she will almost certainly be doing it during her 'nesting' period in the final trimester. But if she goes into labour earlier than expected or the combination of hormones and stress and cravings for pickled food has made her more forgetful than usual, then you could well find yourself tearing around the house gathering up the following:

Night wear

Pyjamas and an old long-length T-shirt or a nightdress and dressing gown she's bought especially for the birth (not the kinky baby-doll gear she's not been able to fit into for the past five months, no matter how much you like seeing her in it).

The birth plan

OK, you will probably be able to recite this easier than your own name, date of birth and PIN by the time you get to the big day – but take a copy of it if either of you have thought to write it down. It may be laughed out of the labour ward or overruled at every stage by the midwife, but at least have a copy to hand and make sure your partner sees that you have it. If there's stuff like this missing at the start of her labour she'll start stressing out – making things tougher for all of you.

Hair brush, toothpaste and brush, hair-bands

You'll be praying she's packed this all in a bath bag already since you're bound to bring the wrong 'scrunchie' – but if she hasn't then scoop up what you can along with shampoo, sanitary towels, soap and make-up – don't panic if you miss stuff, you can always buy toiletries at the hospital.

iPod or CD player

With her chosen playlist of 'Music to Watch Her Waters Break by', this is for her to relax to – so don't be tempted to use this as the ideal opportunity to 'get her into Dylan'. Take spare batteries or have the iPod on charge throughout the entire last month of the pregnancy. Also any books, magazines or personal comforts she requests need to go in the bag too.

Maternity or nursing bra

Hopefully you'll remember what this looks like from the jokes the pair of you made when she first brought it home. Certainly grab a couple of changes of underwear for her at least – and rest assured she'll want her 'big pants', not the thong.

Slippers

Or comfy shoes or flip-flops. Along with the numerous trips to the toilet, your partner may spend much of the initial labour on her feet in order for gravity to help shift the baby further down the birth canal. Hospital floors are cold and not exactly renowned for their bug-free cleanliness, so she'll appreciate you bringing her some appropriate footwear.

Mirror and fan

The mirror is for her to see what's happening down the 'business end'. You'll be the one holding it for her so she can see the head appear. The fan (an electric hand-held one as opposed to a big supporter of your partner) is to cool her down during the labour.

Munchies

Sustenance and energy-providing grub – as well as some stuff that'll just stop her feeling hungry. Take bottled water and red grape juice (the natural sugars will help her deal with the fatigue). Also Lucozade sweets for energy, snack bars or flapjacks for hunger and whatever comfort food she can stomach at the moment – chocolate usually does the trick.

Baby stuff

Oh yes. Knew there was something else. Nappies (newborn size), blanket, size 0 baby grow, vest, warm cardigan, little hat and socks. Basically the stuff that she (and probably you) have been 'cooing' over for the past couple of months.

Use a holdall for all this, or ideally the floral 'overnight bag' she bought months ago, specifically for this moment, and waved in front of you. Remember?

WHAT SHOULD I TAKE ALONG FOR MYSELF?

This is the list you're more likely to need in a hurry:

- **Some cash:** Change for the hospital parking and vending machines, possibly for the telephone too if you can't use your mobile, or you can't get decent reception, or your battery dies. Also handy for buying food or toiletries for you and her if you've forgotten . . .
- **. . . the snacks:** Take your own because you know she'll give you grief if you dare touch anything of hers at this time.

- **Toothbrush, deodorant and change of T-shirt:** Hospitals are hot places and the adrenalin rush coupled with the mad dash of getting to the place means you're going to be humming a little after a while.

- **Camera, camcorder, magazines or game player:** If you're going to film the birth or at least get some photos afterwards then these are essential. As are batteries, or making sure your gadgets are charged. The games and magazines will keep you occupied – or at least divert your mind a little – while your partner is resting.

Expectancy Explained

The Pain Relief Debate

In the build-up to the birth – and during the laying down of the birth plan – you'll need to talk through what pain relief your partner will have during labour – or whether she'll even have it at all. As obstetrician Patrick O'Brien points out, the pain of pregnancy is different for each mother. While many women even get as far as the labour ward with every intention of just saying NO to any drugs, as the pain increases and the duration of the delivery wears on so their resistance wanes. So don't bother saying stuff like, 'But honey, what about the birth plan?' when she starts screaming for anything – anything!!!! – to ease the agony.

HOW CAN I HELP HER DECIDE WHAT PAIN RELIEF TO USE?

Talk to your partner about the various types of pain relief (see Chapter 9) and have her talk to her GP or midwife about the pros and cons of each. It's easy for her to get wrapped up in the many horror stories or old wives' tales thrown her way at this time. If she starts relaying the stuff she's heard from other mums to you, just encourage her to get a definitive, expert answer. Remind her that birth is not some kind of reality TV show challenge in which she has to see how long she can go without getting some help – the pain of childbirth is said to be the most intense pain known to man (well, to woman anyway) and everyone will have their opinion as to what works and what doesn't. In the end, though, she's the one who'll be having this baby so reassure her that you'll support whatever decision she takes.

Did you know?

Papa Knows Her Pain...

Research published by Oxford University Press found that women whose birth partners – including male ones – had learned about the different ways of coping with pain had shorter labours and were less likely to have epidurals.

Do I need any of the drugs?

No, and once you've read up on them you'll know why. But that doesn't stop many an expectant father from having a dabble:

- **Gas and air** is a laugh – though the hospital staff won't think so if they catch you chugging on it.
- **TENS** is far too tempting for any gadget-obsessed male not to try – though don't attempt to sue the manufacturers if it has any Frankenstein-like side effects.
- **Pethidine** – no.
- **Epidural** – definitely not.

Expectancy Explained

Sleepless Nights in Preparation for . . .
More Sleepless Nights

Beginning in the second trimester and lasting well into the third your partner may well develop a snoring habit that you could register on the Richter scale. It's often accompanied by something called sleep apnoea, where she appears to stop breathing – mid-snore – for a short while. It's caused by the baby pushing on her diaphragm – the muscle that controls the chest and lung movements. She'll struggle to get comfy, may choose to rest her bump on a pillow and will be taking plenty of trips to the loo – all of which disruption will at least give you a taster of the nights ahead.

EXPECTANT DADS' EXPERIENCES

The Final Countdown

'Even with a little over five weeks to go, it still doesn't feel real. I know we are going to have a baby and I know that giving birth isn't the easiest thing in the world, but I just can't comprehend that Mel and I are going to be going through this. All the things that being a dad is about excite me – seeing what a mix of Mel and me our baby looks like, teaching him or her various sports, playing silly games with them, teaching them about life while trying not to be too overbearing. Just being a family . . .'
Matthew D

'Right now, with the birth almost imminent, I am worried about Sarah and the baby getting through it all OK. It's not going to be nice seeing her going through so much pain. I know that we'll get to the other side and that it is a natural part of life but I think it's also natural for me to be worried. I'm also nervous about the first time holding the baby as I've not got any experience with babies. I have held a doll in an antenatal class, but I think a real baby might be a bit different! I'm looking forward to being a family together and spending time getting to know our baby.'

Charley G

'Having to work long hours at my job, but wanting to help more around the house and be more supporting to my partner, has been one of the worst sides to the pregnancy. I don't feel that I have spent enough time with her. I clean the flat once a week – before we used to share. I try to get healthy food from the supermarket and I read a story out loud once a week to her and the baby. I don't give her enough massages apparently.'

Paul S

WHY DO I FEEL LIKE RUNNING AWAY RIGHT NOW?

Believe it or not, you're not alone in feeling especially tense right now. If you're experiencing a sudden drop in self-esteem as the birth draws near then this is understandable given the enormity of the task that expectant fathers are about to undertake. Psychologist Russell Hurn says it's because, essentially, you're involved in something that can be incredibly difficult to imagine and conceptualise how to manage.

It's quite common for fathers-to-be to spend moments during the pregnancy questioning their feelings about things. According to Hurn, some focus on their own experiences of a father figure and their own expectations for themselves. If that ideal image in their head is of a perfect father doing everything right and their view of themselves is far removed from this, then the expectant dad is likely to experience a lot of negative thoughts and emotions about themselves. The upshot of all this is stress and self-doubt.

Hurn advises that you talk with your partner about the way you feel about fatherhood. Talk about your own experiences of a dad and what you want to do and feel you can do. Essentially, none of us will be a perfect dad – but we can all aim to be good enough. This involves keeping your child safe, healthy and giving them a good foundation on which they can build their lives.

Preparing for the Big Push

Pregnancy: Weeks 37-40

Through the last month of the pregnancy your baby will be piling on the pounds like a sumo wrestler striving for its best fighting weight. Estimates vary but he or she will possibly add half a pound a week to their little frame so that by the time they leave the uterus and head down – literally if they're the right way round – to the birth canal they could be between 5½ and 9lb (2.5–4kg). Girls tend to weigh less than boys. These are average weights – some may be lighter at birth, some heavier! (If you're expecting twins or triplets don't expect the weight to be shared out evenly (see below). Your baby will now be around 20 inches (50cm) long. Space will be tight in there, so instead of kicking or punching your baby will spend the last few weeks in the womb squirming and 'body-popping'. They'll be able to see, hear, taste, smell and feel.

WE'RE PLAYING THE WAITING GAME, WHAT ELSE CAN I DO?

Without doubt the most frustrating part of the whole pregnancy process is the final few weeks. Your patience may be stretched and your mobile phone may be in meltdown as you deal with the anxious or even false alarm calls from your partner coupled with the well-meaning enquiries from friends and family.

- Change your answerphone message at this point to something along the lines of: 'No sign yet but as soon as the head appears I'll give you a buzz' or possibly something a little less sarcastic.
- Use this time to go through any 'drill' you may have with your partner, such as breathing routines or simply going over the birth plan for the 500th time.
- Load any useful numbers into your phone. The hospital, any friends or relatives you want to call with the good news, Interflora etc.
- Do plan to be doing something on the EDD. I know this sounds odd, but so few first babies arrive on the specified date that you're better off arranging to have a couple of friends round that night to help get over the anticlimax.
- Don't go on the lash. In fact if you're going to be driving your partner to hospital – and it could happen at any hour of the day or night in this final month – you're going to have to steer well clear of the booze for the time being.

AM I REALLY UP TO ATTENDING THE BIRTH?

Your partner won't be the only one having virtual panic attacks during the final stages of pregnancy. Once the stark realisation that you're going to become a father sinks in – and you start finding yourself in areas of a department store you've never previously entered – then you too may start worrying about how you'll fare when it comes to the main event. According to Russell Hurn much of this anxiety is a creation of our own imagination. He says that we have to remember that most things become more frightening for the expectant dad the more he thinks about them.

This becomes a snowball of worry – getting greater and greater – the closer you get to the big event. He suggests anxiety-ridden expectant fathers try this little exercise: Think of some small problem and then say, 'But what if this (bad thing) happened?' – then repeat this again and again. Usually within a few 'what ifs' you are looking at a major disaster. Turn 'what ifs' into 'SO WHATS'. If you are too freaked out during the birth or you pass out, 'so what?'

The key move at this point is to get on to the phone and contact either any of the fathers you met at the antenatal group who will be possibly sharing the same experience, or (even better) some dads who've been through it before.

Expectant dads – and mums – share very similar anxieties before the birth, including:

- Will the baby be healthy?
- How will I cope seeing my partner in pain?
- How will I react during the birth?

The advice of Melvyn Dunstall is to talk to the midwife and health professionals to get feedback on the health of your baby. Express your fears and overcome them by familiarising yourself with things as much as possible, so read up on what's going to happen to her, attend the classes and ask questions. You're going to need to be focused and alert to help out throughout the labour. Getting a few answers may make that a little easier. Accept that you can't take the pain away as such – but deal with her pain by doing all you practically can to comfort and reassure her.

HOW DO THE DIFFERENT TYPES OF PAIN RELIEF DIFFER?

Over 90 per cent of first-time mothers will have some form of pain relief and whether your partner has expressed her preferred drug of choice beforehand or she has a change of heart mid-birth and demands them all, then it's useful for you to know what's on offer and what to say to her when discussing the topic.

TENS machine

Plenty of fathers who've practised fitting a TENS machine to their partner in the days before the EDD and then used one for real during the birth will tell you not to bother with it. To be fair, it gets a bit of a bad press since it's only a basic pain-relief tool that's intended to be used in the very early stages of labour. The 'science' behind it claims that TENS (Transcutaneous Electrical Nerve Stimulation) works by sending small electrical jolts from the power unit, along wires connected to four sticky patches that are applied to your partner's back.

These charges stimulate her body to create its own pain-easing endorphins and so combat the pain of contractions. (Since it's an electrical device it has to be removed again whenever the baby's heart rate needs to be monitored.)

Because the pain will ebb and flow your partner can control the strength of the TENS electrical pulses with a switch. However, TENS works for some mothers and not others. Plenty get ditched within a few minutes of fitting, while others swear it helped them to swear a little less in those early stages.

You can buy one yourself (for example a machine with stick-on pads will cost £49.99 from John Lewis), though many choose to hire them (from £21.95 for six weeks) either through their local health authority or from outlets such as Babytens.net, bodyclock.co.uk or Boots the chemist (www.bootsmaternityrentalproducts.co.uk).

With Boots, for example, you book a TENS unit and it's delivered during the 37th week of pregnancy. It's then returned in a pre-paid envelope after the birth. (Dad job during the birth

– remember not to leave it in the labour ward!) There's a FREE two-week extension to the loan if your baby is late.

Practise attaching the TENS machine to her before she goes into labour and remember, on no account attempt to use it in a birthing pool . . .

Gas and air (Entonox)

A 50/50 oxygen and nitrous oxide mix that she inhales in short gulps through a mask – like Dennis Hopper in *Blue Velvet* – which connects to the hospital's mains supply (or from a gas bottle if it's a planned home birth). Like the TENS it can take a while to have an effect on the pain, but four out of five mothers do have a chug on it at some point during labour.

The Entonox dulls the pain without sending her into a gaseous high – instead the regular draw of breath will relax her, while allowing her to stay in control. She may feel a little nauseous, dizzy and thirsty at times, but there's no risk of harm to her or the baby from taking it.

Pethidine

A morphine-like drug injected into her bum (at her request, of course) that numbs the senses and relaxes her, but leaves her experiencing the sensation of being a little 'drugged up' and not feeling in full control during labour. It's especially useful during a long labour, though the medical team will aim to time it so that they don't give her pethidine if she's close to delivering the baby. Not only would this slow down the birth at just the moment when they're all itching to get it over with, but the pethidine can work its way through the placenta and make the baby drowsy too. Not only will your kid arrive slightly 'stoned', but its rate of breathing and feeding will be slower than normal. If this does happen the medical team have to use another drug on it to reverse the effects.

Epidural

The statistics tell the story with this one. An estimated 95 per cent of women who opt for it get almost total pain relief from having an epidural. The most recent data suggests that up to 60 per cent of first-time mothers opt for an epidural. Why is it such a big hit? Well, it numbs the nerves between the spine and the womb, it has the kick of a mule when it comes to easing the pain of childbirth and if it were we men who had children this would be the compulsory house special, no doubt.

In many hospitals you have to book the epidural in advance. It's a local anaesthetic injected into the base of the spine at a precise point between the vertebrae. As a result it's a specialist task and such marksmanship is in high demand. On the downside, an epidural can be tricky to administer – especially in the throes of some serious contractions. It can take up to 30 minutes to kick in and the dosage may need to be increased if the labour drags on – which will make it tougher for her to push during the contractions. The epidural is very safe – for both your partner and your baby – but there is a small risk of complications,

Expectancy Explained

The Epidural Risk

The mention of needles and the spinal cord understandably causes some concern but any occurrence of epidurals causing severe injury to expectant mothers is extremely rare. Researchers at Bath's Royal United Hospital found the risk of permanent harm to a mother having an epidural was at least as low as 1 in 80,000 and possibly as low as 1 in 300,000.

including a drop in the mother's blood pressure, which may need to be countered with more drugs, loss of bladder control (though that may well occur anyway) and the possibility – about a 1 in 200 risk – of her suffering from a severe headache for about a week after the birth.

WATER BIRTHS

One in 10 women opt for a water birth, which is in itself one of the most common forms of natural pain relief. Whether at home or at the hospital the warm water will relax her muscles and support her body – so much so that just 24% of first-time mothers who had water births needed pain-relieving drugs. (It's 50% for non-bath births.).

Hypno-birthing

Some mothers-to-be take hypnotherapy courses prior to the birth or else rely on the breathing techniques they've learned through their antenatal classes in order to have as natural a birth as possible.

Regardless of which options your partner goes for you can help her along the way. Encouraging her to focus on her breathing – and ideally take her mind off the pain slightly – is something you can do. Instead of simply standing there saying 'breathe' though, join in with her. Practise the breathing technique prior to labour with her – simply drawing in deep breaths through the nose and out through the mouth. Practise getting into a rhythm doing it along with her. It'll seem odd doing this at home, but on the day simple acts like this not only help her feel in control but reassure her that you're there supporting her as best you can.

WHAT ELSE CAN I DO TO HELP EASE HER PAIN?

OK, you won't be administering the drugs yourself, but there are plenty of moves an expectant dad can use to help her through the labour:

- **Rubbing**. Firm pressure wherever she demands it – and reassuring words from the early stages – will help stimulate her body to release 'feel-good' hormones, or endorphins. A little 'shiatsu' at this point can go a long way. Practise your back-rub technique in advance and be prepared to get down on all fours while she kneels down and rests – possibly rocking back and forth – on you.

- **Cuddling**. Assuring her that everything is going to be OK and that you're there for her will ease her anxieties – and yours. But beware, while this may help her at first, once she's in 'the zone' she may not want to be touched at all. Don't take this personally – she'll be focused on getting the labour over with and your baby out.

- **Cooling**. Take along a bottle of chilled water or ensure your partner has a constant supply of it.

- **Coaching**. Encourage her to groan, moan or scream – whatever she feels helps. Don't think you're wasting your time. Research shows that when a woman has someone supportive with her during labour, she gives birth more quickly and easily than if she doesn't have continuous support.

There will be blood. Prepare yourself as best you can and keep yourself in good shape through the birth by drinking water and grabbing a snack when you can, and don't forget to offer your partner one. If you do feel as if you're going to pass out – and it's rare that men do at the birth – don't worry. Just get yourself back together as soon as possible, you've still got a role to play. Frankly, the midwives have seen it all and are all geared up for it, and a hospital is probably the best place of all to pass out in.

I'M WORRIED ABOUT WHAT THE BABY WILL BE BORN LIKE, IS THIS NORMAL?

Concern about how healthy your child will be is something that both parents share throughout the pregnancy – though they may avoid speaking about it for fear of upsetting the other. It's a reaction that psychologists believe often stems from a misunderstanding or preconception. Yes, there are always problems for some and they cannot be eliminated completely, but the risks are very low. Talk to a health professional about the level of risk and your concerns – especially if you don't want to burden your partner with them. Then compare the facts and risk factors to your daily life. Hurn suggests that when you look at the facts you will probably find you are more likely to be involved in a car accident than experience birth defects. Then ask yourself how much you worry about driving, or crossing the road after a few drinks, or climbing a ladder at home?

Hurn concedes that he, like many expectant fathers, was worried during his partner's pregnancy about the risk of Down's syndrome. He has since found that his chief concern – which was not so much for the child or his partner but an admittedly selfish one of how he would manage the situation – isn't uncommon. However, it is something you will never know unless it happens and can never really plan for.

WILL I BE WITH HER ALL THE TIME?

Certainly if you don't pass out you will. If she has to go for a caesarean you will be asked to 'scrub up' and wear surgical clothing, but you'll be asked to leave her side only if there's a major problem. Otherwise you'll simply be asked to stay close, be supportive and get out of the way if needs be. Be prepared for a labour that could last 10, 20 or more hours, though. If she's resting you may want to get some fresh air, phone friends and family with updates or simply take a break and get your head together. If you need to go home to fetch anything or make arrangements you can alert the ward sister or midwife and ask them to contact you if you need to dash back.

WHO ELSE WILL BE AT THE BIRTH?

For a hospital birth it'll be a midwife, or possibly a spate of midwives depending on how many shifts your partner's labour stretches through.

If you're having a home birth there'll be at least one, often two, midwives present. Your home will have been assessed beforehand to see if it's suitable but if the midwife feels that a home birth cannot be carried out safely she'll call ahead to the hospital.

At the hospital, so long as the whole thing is going smoothly, you'll probably find that you'll be the one comforting your partner as her contractions intensify, while the midwife on shift checks in on you every now and again.

The midwife at the hospital won't necessarily be one that your partner's met with or dealt with on her previous visits. Also, different midwives have different approaches – so be prepared for some contradictions in the messages they're giving you. Be sure to communicate your partner's concerns to the midwife. Don't be afraid to ask what's going on or to request whatever your partner may want, such as water or a snack.

The key is to avoid having your partner getting stressed out – and ideally to stick to your chosen birth plan as closely as possible. Voice any concerns you have but be aware that you won't be the only couple there having a baby that day. Also, birth can be a long and extremely boring process for much of the time and it's easy to get frustrated with things that are beyond your control.

Remember your role. You're there to keep her company and help the time pass as easily as possible – not to try and rush things along. If you're not happy about the way you've been treated make a note of names and times and deal with it in your own time after everything has settled down.

The cast

At around the point when your partner begins pushing with all her might then you may find that the room around her bed becomes a lot less spacious. Possible cast members you'll see are:

The obstetrician:

The pregnancy specialist doctor who may do anything from popping his head around the door to say 'Hi', to ignoring you both completely, or else spending an unnerving amount of time seemingly obsessed with your partner and her womb. In this last case it's most likely because of some complications surrounding her pregnancy or the labour. If there are any problems during the pregnancy this is the person your midwife or GP will consult with.

The anaesthetist:

The man or woman who'll administer the epidural if your partner decides to have one. It's a skilled task – the needle must be accurately placed in the 'epidural' space around the lumbar region of her back. Your partner won't be on best form at this point, to put it mildly, as she'll have been in labour for hours, with the pain peaking, and may be angry with herself for having to go down this route. Get in there and support her as best you can – especially if she has a thing about needles. Face your partner, hold her hands, comfort her and aim to keep her as calm as possible while the anaesthetist goes to work. These people are very cool under fire. Be sure to send them a big thank-you card or buy them a very large drink once it's all over.

The midwife:

What seems like a revolving door policy will be in operation while your partner is in the final throes of labour. Staff will come and go – usually snaffling equipment like the foetal heart monitor or cardiotocograph (CTG) machine to take to another mother-to-be. This 'Piccadilly Circus' feel to the labour ward is one reason why some women opt for the home birth option. Along with the CTG, another piece of kit you may see wheeled in as the delivery of your baby gets really close is a trolley-like device with an overhead heater. It has a platform on it about waist height. It's here that the midwife or paediatrician will put your baby, briefly, after it's born in order to give it a quick check over, to wipe away any mucus from its mouth and nose and even to give it a little oxygen to get its breathing started.

The paediatrician:

Another specialist, this time one dealing with babies and sick children. Don't be alarmed by their presence though; it's their job to check over all babies born on their patch before they're taken home (though apparently nowadays more and more midwives undertake the examination of the newborn – the paediatrician may be called if there are any problems).

Medical students:

They've all got to learn somehow and you may well find your-self sat in a room with your partner – swaying between pain and exhaustion – and a student who's seemingly just there for the ride. They'll come in handy for fetching drinks and offering sympathetic smiles if nothing else.

How I can be sure I'll be at the birth?

Short of having a caesarean booked, there's no way you can absolutely, unreservedly, without any doubt, ensure that your first ever appointment with your newborn boy or girl will be timed to coincide perfectly. But the chances are that IF you want to be at the birth of your child then you will make it.

That's the beauty of a woman going into labour – it can last for hours, usually giving you ample time to leave work, or the pub, and be there in time for the head to appear. (Best not mention this little benefit to her when you arrive though.)

Just to be on the safe side, however, be sure to do the following:

Take all calls:

Even ones on your work phone. You may have both agreed that she should call you on your mobile phone once she goes into labour, but that plan may go out the window if she's in the throes of labour or if someone else is calling you on her behalf.

Clear the diary:

Get used to making sacrifices to your social life now – there'll be plenty more to come in the future. Let your mate have your season ticket for the Gunners/United/Spearmint Rhino for the next few weeks, or at least avoid going to any away games. Negotiate with work to avoid being sent anywhere long-haul over the next few weeks (unless you're a pilot this should be manageable).

Fuel up the car:

Calling out the AA to not only top up an empty tank but also help deliver your baby in your stranded vehicle won't endear you to your partner nor do much for your upholstery.

Load up on coins:

If you're going to drive her to the hospital when she goes into labour, find out what the situation is regarding the hospital car park well beforehand – ideally during the antenatal class stage or if you get to do a tour of the hospital.

Check in with base:

Call her regularly through the day and let her know when you're going to be out of phone range to avoid her becoming anxious if she can't get hold of you.

Stay sober:

Obviously.

EXPECTANT DADS' EXPERIENCES

Waiting Game

'Those last couple of weeks were the worst of the pregnancy for both of us. We argued a lot as I struggled to deal with the workload while also helping around the house. I started to worry that things would go wrong. Her back was playing up but she wouldn't complain about it. Instead she'd go into herself. We brought a pillow for her to rest her bump upon to make things a little easier and I'd rub her back too, but the worst thing was I was powerless to do anything to speed things up.'

Paul S

CAN CURRY OR SEX HELP MOVE THINGS ALONG A BIT?

So the theory goes. The best explanation for this is that hot, spicy foods can provoke bowel movements that in turn give the uterus a nudge and may bring on labour. Alternatively, nipple stimulation (hers, naturally) is said to trigger the release of the hormone oxytocin, which in turn may get your baby moving. You can decide which of these two courses you may want to follow.

Expectancy Explained

What's Worrying Her – The Baby isn't Moving

Just as your partner has got used to the rave that kicks off inside her stomach at random points of the day, so your baby will start to play the first of many frightening and unintentional tricks upon you. 'Freezing' is one of them. More often in the final weeks of the pregnancy – when space is tight – your baby won't be able to move around so much. According to Dr Patrick O'Brien, your partner may worry that a lack of movement signals a possible problem. Although most mums-to-be should feel around 10 movements a day from about week 20 onwards, this will vary and often, if she's distracted, she may not even notice your nipper's womb-based aerobics. O'Brien suggests you tell her to lie down with her hands on her stomach for a while. If your baby has a lot of amniotic fluid around it then the movements can be harder to detect – trying this should reassure her. If she's still concerned then there's no harm in contacting her midwife or phoning the hospital – take her along and hold her hand while they check her out.

HOW WILL I KNOW SHE'S GOING INTO LABOUR?

Trying to cut things as fine as possible between taking time off work and attending the birth? Or simply aiming to make yourself scarce? Well, you may get a 'heads up' that your baby has had enough and now wants out through a series of signs.

Your partner will have been warned about them but they'll most likely come as a bit of a shock to you. As ever, don't panic – your partner only wants to see one wailing mess in the next 48 hours – and remember that the birth itself is still a long way off (at least until you get to the hospital, you hope).

Obviously there's a good chance you may experience a few false alarms too – be patient and don't start saying things to her like 'crying wolf again, eh?' if you find yourself rushing to the hospital for the umpteenth time.

Drop and engage

A bit like 'lock and load' in that your baby has moved into the chamber and is ready to be fired. This is especially prominent in first-time mums and involves the baby dropping into the pelvic area a week or so before labour begins. It causes the baby to press on her bladder – leading to even more frequent trips to the loo.

Dashing to the loo

A few days before her labour starts a woman's body releases prostaglandin, which can sometimes prompt a sudden attack of diarrhoea as a precursor to going into labour. You may have a 'sympathy' bout of this too on hearing the news.

Bloody show

Not in the drama sense, though there may be plenty of that too. No, this is a leak of a mucous bloody discharge from her cervix out of her vagina. Not something you personally are likely to come across, but a trigger for her all the same. If the description of this alone has you feeling a little squeamish then you're really going to struggle through the next chapter.

Bigger, bolder contractions

During these last few weeks those Braxton Hicks practice contractions will get stronger – it'll be easy for her to mistake them for labour pains, because that's what they'll become.

Those contractions – the tightening and then relaxing of her uterus muscles – will start to become more frequent, more regular and last longer. She may well have been able to walk around to ease the Braxton Hicks contractions, but once they start becoming real contractions she'll know the difference. They are, by all accounts, more like period cramps with added backache twinges. Once they're lasting for around 30 seconds or more then she's in labour. You could fuss around with a stopwatch at this point – if you're actually there – but there's a good chance she'll make it clear that she's in labour as she begins swearing at you and continues to do so with greater velocity and variety of vocabulary until your baby is finally born.

Breaking waters

If everything you think you know about childbirth so far is what you've learned from TV then you'll know that 'her waters breaking' is a pretty significant moment. It's when membranes – the fluid sac inside her – rupture. She – and you – may notice a 'gush' of fluid, though this doesn't happen every time. Otherwise she may notice a leak of the amniotic fluid (the liquid protecting your baby), which may be clear or a pinkish colour. Your baby will be OK, but things are definitely moving on now.

Check the water:

A word of warning. Midwife Dunstall advises couples to ring up the labour ward if the water is green/black. The most likely cause of this is the baby has opened its bowels in the uterus and the staining is caused by meconium (baby's first poo). The presence of meconium may indicate that the baby is distressed.

If any of these occur on your watch, you may want to cancel tonight's attendance at the pub quiz.

Did you know?

The Push Present . . .

One final 'essential' for you to buy, though not in the company of your partner, is the push present or 'Mother's Little Hamper' as some call it. It's a birth gift for your partner. It could be flowers or something like jewellery to commemorate the occasion or else it could be something she's not had for a while – chocolate, champagne, full-strength cider.

WHAT DO I DO WHEN SHE GOES INTO LABOUR?

If she's experiencing any number of the 'signs' outlined above then you can help her time the period between her contractions to see if it's time to get her to hospital or not. Don't be afraid to call the hospital at any time of the day or night – the maternity ward doesn't operate a nine-to-five policy only when it comes to births. The sooner you prepare the hospital for your arrival by calling ahead and letting them know how close your partner is to giving birth, the better.

It's not unusual for pregnant mothers to be sent home from hospital because it's too early in their labour for the maternity ward to provide a bed for her. You obviously want to ensure she gets there in plenty of time – if nothing else to avoid delivering it yourself – to avoid being refused entry check for the following signs:

- Are her contractions lasting between 40 seconds and a minute in length?
- Are they not easing when she changes position or tries walking around?
- Is she finding it hard or completely unable to talk during a contraction?

Answer yes to all these and she's definitely *not* having false ones now. Call the hospital maternity ward (have the phone number next to your home phone and stored in both yours and her mobile phones).

Tell them how far apart the contractions are – if they're between five and 10 minutes they'll almost definitely want her to come in.

HOW DO HELL DO I 'TIME HER CONTRACTIONS'?

Contractions are like a mix between a really bad period and constipation – she may say this is what she's feeling to you. The pain can start in her lower back and move toward the stomach, or just linger around as a pain in her backside – she may say this is what she's thinking of you. To start with they will probably last around 30 seconds and occur every 15 minutes. To time them start counting from the beginning of one contraction to the beginning of the next – she'll obviously need to tell you when the feeling kicks in. (Write them down, it's easier). As things progress so the gap gets shorter – while the pain bit gets longer. You may be asked 'How far apart are the contractions?'

You won't get deducted anything for a wrong answer but giving the medical staff a rough idea may help them prioritise things.

EXPECTANT DADS' EXPERIENCES

Going into Labour

'I was using a contraction timer on the internet – for about 16 hours the contractions were getting steadily less, then about two in the morning (after 16 hours or so) they started getting longer again – we called the hospital and they said it was normal – but I called again and a midwife said we could come in for a check. I'm glad we did as when we arrived and my wife was put on the baby monitor, we could see the baby's heart rate dropping with every contraction – that was when we really started to get worried and were happy to be at the hospital. Also, after the internal exam, there were some huge contractions that left my wife shaking and crying in pain. That was rough.'

Tom L

Should I drive her or get an ambulance?

Only call an ambulance in an absolute emergency. Although labour has begun, that baby won't arrive for quite some time yet. Women do drive themselves to hospital when in labour. It does happen. In the USA one woman was even given a speeding ticket while doing it. But it's not really part of the whole birthing experience that anyone would recommend. Instead, if you're there and you do drive, you've got to take her – ideally in the back seat if she can get in OK, and with her belt on.

On arrival at the hospital take your partner straight to the Maternity Department before trying to find somewhere to park. A midwife will take her to be examined and find out how close you now are to becoming a father.

10

Your Child is Born

The Stages of Labour

During the birth your baby will twist into a position so that it pushes down on the opening of your partner's uterus – that opening is called the cervix. Labour itself comes in a series of stages. The first is called the 'latent phase' by the white coats and refers to when her contractions may have started but her cervix has not dilated (not to four centimetres anyway).

Once four centimetres has been reached then the midwife will note the time because your partner is now deemed to be in 'active' labour. The contractions will cause her cervix to widen (or dilate as the midwife puts it) until eventually there's about a 10-centimetre opening – she should now have a strong urge to push your baby out. However, it sometimes may need some assistance in the form of forceps or a ventouse (see below).

Of course, there's the chance that your partner may have chosen to have a caesarean birth. Or she may have been advised to, despite hours in labour trying to have a natural birth, because it's deemed the best option if the baby is becoming distressed.

Once the baby is born it's the third stage. At this point the placenta – your baby's oxygen and nutrition 'backpack' for the last nine months – is expelled by the uterus contracting down. This may take up to an hour to occur naturally but in most cases this stage is 'managed' by the midwife – which means the mother is given an injection immediately after the birth containing drugs that stimulate the uterus to contract. The midwife then applies traction on the cord to bring out the placenta and membranes.

BUT WHAT IF SHE STARTS GIVING BIRTH AND I'M THE ONLY ONE THERE?

Here's something you may think only occurs on TV. It's a major fear for many an expectant dad – though, armed with the right knowledge, it needn't be. If your partner goes into labour and you're unable to get her to hospital or contact the midwife in time for them to assist with a home birth, then you're going to have to deliver the baby yourself. With first-time mums this is very unlikely but very occasionally it does happen. In the event of you and your partner being one such rare couple then don't run around shouting for someone (God knows who?) to fetch hot water and towels. Instead midwife Melvyn Dunstall suggests you do the following:

- If it looks as if baby is coming call 999 and ask for an ambulance. Tell them your partner is in full-blown labour and there's no health professional present. That way it gets logged as an emergency.

- Then ring the hospital maternity unit – most units will despatch a community midwife to attend ASAP. If you're worried, ask the midwife to stay on the phone. You will need to calmly describe to the midwife what is happening.

- Get your partner as comfortable as possible. Do grab some towels or blankets and place them around her on the floor. These will soak up the amniotic fluid and blood. Anything absorbent will do the trick. Keep a couple of towels to one side to wipe the baby with and wrap it in.

- Wedge a pillow or rolled-up towel beneath your partner's lower back so that she's not lying completely flat – this prevents the weight of the baby pressing on veins and hindering her blood supply.

- Encourage her to push with the contractions, breathe calmly and not to hold her breath, and keep reassuring her that everything will be OK.

- Let her know when you see the baby's head emerging. Check to see that the umbilical cord is not wrapped around your baby's neck. If so, release it, being careful not to tug on the cord.

- Place your hands under the baby's head to help guide it out – don't try to pull it. If you can, use a towel to catch your baby (with the next contraction it will come fairly quickly) since it'll be coated with fluid, blood and delivery 'goo'.

- Wrap your baby in the towel and rub him or her on the back to dry them and start them crying – this is good as it'll help them take their first breaths too.

- Hand it over to the missus (nothing like getting in the habit of doing this early). Midwives insist on skin-to-skin contact with the mother almost immediately as the best way of avoiding the baby getting cold. Most babies, if placed on their mother's chest with breasts exposed, will also instinctively latch on to the breast and begin feeding.

- **DO NOT CUT THE CORD.** If the placenta is delivered leave it intact, and the midwife/paramedic will deal with it. These deliveries are called BBAs (born before arrival in hospital) by those abbreviation-loving hospital folk. Often when the midwife attends a BBA and all is well the mother and baby will stay at home, but if there are any concerns then the midwife may suggest they go off to the hospital for a checkup.

WHAT HAPPENS WHEN WE REACH THE HOSPITAL?

If you haven't just delivered the baby yourself and instead are taking your partner into hospital because she's in the early throes of labour then you'll need to report to the maternity reception to 'check in' your partner. Then you'll head off to a room on the labour ward where the midwife can carry out an internal examination, looking to see how wide your partner's cervix has dilated and so gauge how close she is to actually giving birth.

Your partner's blood pressure and temperature will be checked too. The midwife will also listen to the baby's heart rate with either a handheld Doppler or Pinard stethoscope. If there are any concerns about the baby's heartbeat your partner will be wired up to a device that sounds a little like the vidiprinter they used to use on *Grandstand* to give out football results – called the foetal heart monitor. The midwife then checks on the baby's 'latest scores' throughout the labour.

HOW DO THEY 'INDUCE' LABOUR AND WHY?

When the midwife finally says 'enough is enough' – especially likely if your partner is in the 42nd or 43rd week – then she or he will use one of a number of ploys to hasten the arrival of your child.

These include a **sweep of the membranes,** where the midwife dons a rubber glove and sweeps her fingers across your partner's cervix (don't try this at home) in a bid to release the labour-provoking hormones (prostaglandins). This is done before labour has begun to get things started.

Induction – jump-starting the labour – usually comes as a great relief to an overdue mother (also the baby, no doubt). More often than not your partner will be asked to come into the hospital at a certain date and time. Then a gel or pessary is applied to do what the sweep does. Once the decision to induce is made then your partner won't leave the hospital until that little lass or fella has appeared. As a result inductions are more likely to require a caesarean section too.

Breaking the waters. For this they may use an ARM. Not a real one. ARM stands for Artificially Rupturing the Membrane and involves using a probe to pierce the amniotic sac your baby is living in and so causing your partner's waters to break. This will only be done if the cervix is at least four centimetres dilated and she's experiencing contractions.

Remember also, prostaglandins are the same hormones that occur naturally in sperm, so **having sex** in the final weeks of pregnancy can stir things up – this doesn't mean there and then on the labour ward though.

WHAT'S MY ROLE DURING LABOUR?

The labour pains and contractions will continue to come and go in waves. Your role at this point – aside from remembering the overnight bag and its multitude of contents – is to:

Be her crutch

Not an ideal turn of phrase at this point, admittedly, but you can provide her with physical support as she walks around the ward or just needs someone to lean on as she stands up. Encourage her to do so too. This style of 'active birth' can speed up the labour and may be more comfortable for her than lying on her back.

Rub her up

Massage, if nothing else, will take her mind off things a little. Be on hand with the back rubs. For more intense contractions she may insist you press your thumbs into her back, applying a bit of acupressure that'll help ease the pain.

Keep her on the ball

Some midwives will wheel out a huge rubber fitness (Swiss) ball for your partner to sit on and even gently bounce on. *Gently* mind – not Space Hopper-like bounds around the room. Doing this encourages the baby to follow the gravitational pull down the birth canal and opens your partner's pelvis. You'll help by holding her at the hips and making sure she doesn't fall off.

Help her into labour positions

Impress her with your knowledge of all things prenatal by suggesting she try some of the following moves to relieve the pain or speed things up. Be prepared to be sworn at despite your help, and do back off if she tells you to. Some women often find their own way of coping with the pain. Positions she should try include:

- Standing up and leaning on the bed or you.
- Kneeling down and leaning on the seat of a chair.
- Kneeling – with one leg raised – to shift the position of her pelvis.

- Getting on all fours (help her here by placing a blanket on the floor and supporting her).
- Rocking her hips as much as she can to get the baby moving.
- Walking around – encourage her to be mobile as an upright position will help.

Expectancy Explained

What's the Big Deal with 'Breathing' Exercises?

It's a question that may have been gnawing away at you since the antenatal classes. A huge amount of emphasis is placed upon how your partner should breathe when having contractions. The thinking behind the rhythmic breathing techniques the midwives teach you both is that by timing the inhale-and-exhale you can maximise the effectiveness of your efforts. If you've ever lifted dumb-bells – properly – you'll have some idea of how you're supposed to inhale deeply to fill the muscles and blood with oxygen then exhale with force in order to give the 'lift' – or in the case of labour, the 'push' – added momentum.

That's how breathing is meant to work for your partner at this point – just swap the dumb-bells for an eight-pound wriggling bundle of baby firmly wedged into the vagina and I'm sure you get the idea.

Some touchline coaching on your part will come in very handy here. You may be met with reactions such as 'I AM FUCKING BREATHING!' but persevere. You need to help her focus on how she draws her breath because:

- Encouraging slow breathing out enables relaxation. Holding a breath causes tension.

- If she's taking too many short, frequent breaths she runs the risk of hyperventilating.
- If she's not breathing in time with her contractions – exhaling as she contracts her abdominal muscles – she may find it harder to push her baby through.

Try breathing with her, offering words of encouragement, and ensure both your partner and yourself have plenty to drink. Isotonic sports drinks like Lucozade are especially good if she can stomach them. Even in the birthing pool. The labour ward and maternity suites are especially hot so that newborn babies are kept in the 'womb' style to which they're accustomed. This heat will dehydrate the pair of you though, so fill up on water when you can.

Aside from the breathing tips your partner may now be opting for the first in that series of painkillers on offer, the Entonox (gas and air). The drugs, heat and stress can cause some nausea and occasional vomiting (for your partner) so scan the room for something for her to spew into if needs be.

HOW DO I FIND OUT WHAT'S GOING ON?

Ask, ask, ask. All the time. If you're unsure of what's happening then your partner will most likely be pretty much in the dark too – and a lot more worried. For her sake demand some feedback if you feel you need it. The midwife and support staff will keep regular checks on your partner and the baby throughout the labour and will tell you if they have any concerns. If she has stipulated in her birth plan which painkillers she wants then the hospital should have these ready to administer or the anaesthetist who performs the epidural injection will be called upon to do the deed. It's crucial at this point that you relay any of your partner's worries to the midwife while also doing all you can to help the medics do the best for your partner. Vital decisions affecting the health and safety of her and the baby may need to be taken quickly – it pays if you can arm yourself with all the facts you need to know beforehand.

Expectancy Explained

Prepare for Poo

The experience of birth may be many things to different couples – joyous and bountiful, traumatic and hellish – but one thing it certainly is not is dignified. You're going to see a side to your partner never previously revealed. This will most likely leave you in jaw-dropping awe of her ability to bring your child into the world while experiencing pain the likes of which no man will ever know or suffer. However, the bit that'll never leave your mind is if she poos herself. It doesn't happen to all mothers but it can occur at any moment as her entire internal system seemingly goes into meltdown. It may happen on the bed or in the birthing pool as she pushes or struggles to control the contractions. Your role at this point is to ignore it completely. A midwife will clean it up in a very brisk matter-of-fact manner, but otherwise never mention it and certainly don't film it . . .

NOW SHE'S BEING TOLD TO PUSH, IS THIS IT?

Yep, at this stage your baby is on the way. Usually at about the moment you think it can't go on any more – your partner's pain, your anxiety, the heat, the breathing, the drugs, the contractions . . . then she begins, on the midwife's instruction, a series of big pushes. Her body more or less steers her along as the desire to push can be overwhelming, breathing a couple of deep breaths as the closer contractions start and she pushes down. Your partner may now be crouching or squatting to give more power to the push and let gravity help out too. You may be asked to support her from behind by holding her under her arms – equally you may be ordered to get out of the way.

At this point many an expectant dad does what comes naturally. Gently telling her how much you love her may seem like the most random and inappropriate instruction to pass on to you but plenty of dads find that this moment is often the first time they've said it in front of a crowd of strangers – don't be surprised if this and similar words of encouragement pour forth. Things are reaching a climax and as her pain and discomfort peaks so both you and she will see that the end is in sight. Don't hold back! She needs you now more than ever to be a rock for her.

If you're standing at the 'business end' or simply holding a mirror there for her to see what's happening then you're going to witness a magical moment. Not every expectant dad is up to seeing the 'crowning' – the moment the top of your baby's head appears at the vaginal opening – but for the many that do it's reported as something they'll never forget. Some dads, on the other hand, can't handle this moment at all. Your partner will most likely want to give one almighty 'heave' at this point, though the midwife may instruct her to ease up once the top half of the head is visible – to push slowly and gently to give the skin and muscles around the perineum (the area between her vagina and back passage) a moment to stretch without tearing.

The harsh truth for the squeamish dad is that with birth there will be blood. There will be a whole load of pain – for her. And you're not going to enjoy a great deal of this either. Finally, witnessing your partner undergo this traumatic ordeal at the culmination of the past God knows how many hours will, without doubt, cement the admiration you hold for her and all of womankind . . . well, the ones that have kids, at least. If you're overjoyed at this point don't be afraid to let it out.

EXPECTANT DADS' EXPERIENCES

The Birth

'Sarah's waters broke at 7 a.m., contractions started about 2 p.m. and the second stage started about midnight. Joe was born at 2.15 a.m. and the midwives left at 5 a.m. That means that it was only technically 12 hours but all went on for nearly 24. The home birth was tough for Sarah without any pain relief but we'd do the same again as it was great being at home rather than in hospital. The toughest bit for me was seeing her in so much pain. I wasn't squeamish and although I had worried about this before it wasn't an issue. We were lucky that everything went to plan and there were no complications and no intervention was required. I think that it was important to have learned about the birth in advance and to have also discussed the birth plan. I watched some births on YouTube and this helped me to overcome squeamishness and feel more prepared. I don't think that most expectant fathers would want to, but it helped me.'

Charley G

Your to-do list during labour

- Be there: hold hands, wipe face with a damp cloth (her face), provide water and words of encouragement.
- Relay any questions to the midwife if your partner is too anxious or overwhelmed by her labour to speak up.

- Massage her lower back and help her change position or get comfortable.
- Support her decisions regarding birth method, painkillers, poor choice of background music throughout.
- Breathe along with her to help keep a pattern during the contractions.
- Tell your partner what's happening as the baby is born – be prepared to have to watch and commentate on the delivery if she wants you to.
- **Do not** at this moment decide to: run away from the ward shouting, 'I'm not cut out for fatherhood'; say stuff like 'Is that meant to look like that?'; or imply in any way that your partner should deal with the pain and get a move on because otherwise you're going to miss *Match of the Day*.

What's an episiotomy?

You're going to wish you hadn't asked this, or else you're going to cross your legs and wince a lot during the next few sentences. Sometimes the skin of the perineum – the outer lining of the vagina – cannot stretch enough for the baby's head to pass through. In which case the midwife or doctor will ask your partner's permission to administer a local anaesthetic to the area and then perform a small surgical cut to make the opening bigger.

This may later be stitched up or left to heal naturally – though the midwives I spoke to confirm that it's rare for a woman to refuse suturing after this. Sometimes more serious tears occur that the medical staff will treat immediately after the birth.

If you're still reading, then the episiotomy is often carried out in conjunction with either the use of forceps to pull your baby out, or a ventouse – or both. Again, if you've a ringside seat, this is going to hurt you just watching it. Imagine how your partner is feeling and be prepared for her to tear your hand to shreds while you look away vowing never to attend a birth again. If nothing else deters you from pestering your partner for sex within a day or two of the birth then perhaps a quick recollection of this will be enough.

And a ventouse?

You may have seen or heard tell of the ventouse extraction or a forceps delivery from the antenatal class. Back then they may have been referred to as tools used for 'assisted deliveries'. In reality they're pretty gruesome contraptions. The ventouse – its name means a cupping glass – is actually a metallic or rubber cap that is shaped a little like the end of a plumber's sink plunger and does a similar kind of job. By creating a vacuum beneath the cap and attaching it to the visible crown of your baby's head, the obstetrician may use the ventouse to drag your child from its mother, with the resultant effect of leaving it with a cone-shaped red swelling on the top of its head for a few days (called a chignon), but thankfully no other major side effects.

I know what forceps are . . . but why?

In the event of the ventouse not being up to the job then the forceps will be called for. These look like two large tongs and, like the plumber's plunger in the previous paragraph, tongs are pretty much what they are. These are inserted into your partner's vagina and placed around the baby's cheeks and jaw (feel free to read that again if you're struggling to believe at this point). Then, the forceps are used to gently guide the baby's head out of the birth canal. Around one in eight regular (non-caesarean) births are carried out using these tools.

Won't this cause permanent damage to her?

If your partner has an assisted birth or episiotomy she's a lot more likely to suffer from soreness and bruising after the birth – along with some pain and numbness in her nether regions and perhaps a problem with incontinence for a while. Again, be sensitive to this, especially when your mind drifts off to thoughts of sex, and don't be surprised if she wants to take things slowly at first or has to stop during sex because of the discomfort. In time things will heal – just as in time your baby will get over that crying phase. But it can take months or longer. Sleep and sex are among the many sacrifices you're going to have to make before and after the birth to some extent. If you're feeling hard done by then don't think that your partner having a caesarean instead will make the postnatal nookie come any quicker either.

WHAT IF SHE'S HAVING A CAESAREAN, DO I GO ALONG TOO?

Around 26 per cent of babies are born by caesarean or 'c-section' in the UK. Caesarean means the baby is delivered after an incision is made in your partner's abdomen and uterus at around the position of her bikini line, not that you'll have seen her bikini of late.

Because it's a form of surgery you'll have to scrub and gownup like the medical team. You'll be able to stand beside your partner and comfort her and see the baby for yourself just as you would a natural birth. Be ready with the goalkeeper's gloves too – you may be the first to hold the baby when it's delivered by c-section while your partner is being stitched up by the surgeon.

Your partner may be having an elective caesarean (13.2 per cent are), which means she's chosen to have a birth in this way and so will know exactly what day the baby will arrive on. The midwife may have advised her to go for an elective caesarean for any number of reasons, including a risk to her or the baby through having a natural birth – for instance if the position of the baby or the placenta makes a caesarean a safer option, or possibly if your partner is suffering with pre-eclampsia – or the fact that it's twins or triplets or more!

Alternatively, your partner may have to undergo an emergency caesarean – usually because the baby is in some distress, or there are complications such as the umbilical cord collapsing or becoming wrapped around your baby's neck, or the failure of your partner's cervix to dilate fully. This can be a last resort after your partner has spent many hours in labour and though she may hate the thought of not being able to have her baby the way she wants it, the advice of the medical staff will be to have a caesarean immediately.

She may already have had an epidural or a similar type of local anaesthetic called a 'spinal', or she may be given one there and then. She'll be taken into theatre and a screen will be placed across her chest. She'll be awake throughout, although the anaesthetic will prevent her feeling anything too severe when the surgeons perform the caesarean. On average it takes about 10 minutes to deliver a baby in this way. Your baby then needs to be checked, measured, wiped and weighed before being handed over to you while the surgeon carries out stage three of the birth, the removal of the placenta.

Another common complication to occur that can lead to a c-section delivery is when the baby is born bum and feet first instead of head first. This is called a 'breech birth'. Until around 32 weeks into the pregnancy about 20 per cent of babies lie in this position. By the time of birth most have moved into the 'head-first' spot.

While one in five UK births are caesarean sections, around one in five of those are for breech births. The obstetrician may attempt to move the baby into the head-first (or cephalic) position manually, literally by pushing your partner's bump around (known in the trade as an external cephalic version or ECV). But there may come a point when a caesarean is deemed to be the safer option. Your partner may still be able to give birth to your baby normally while it's in the breech position – if so an epidural and the forceps are both more likely to be used.

Expectancy Explained

What's Worrying Her . . . The Smell of Your Fear

Fathers who are anxious during a caesarean operation may increase the pain experienced by the mother. Studies from the University of Bath and Imperial College London carried out on women who'd elected for a caesarean birth found that the way that their 'birth partners' (that's you) felt during the operation related to the levels of fear and anxiety experienced by the mother. This increased the amount of pain the woman felt immediately after the operation, which could affect her immediate recovery as well as potentially influencing other factors such as breast-feeding and bonding with the child.

How long will it take for her to recover from a caesarean?

You've not been wearing those scrubs for comic effect; she's just undergone major surgery, remember. As a result your partner will need some serious rest and recuperation afterwards. She may have to stay in hospital for several days. She'll certainly have stitches running across her abdomen, which will make moving tricky, driving impossible, lifting forbidden, sex out of the question (again), and your trapeze act will have to take a back seat for a while. Full recovery from a caesarean can take six weeks. In that time the most she'll be able to do is to feed your baby. You as a new dad are going to have to be doubly hands-on at doing stuff around the house once she and the baby come home.

Did you know?

Using Caesars to Cut with . . .

The term caesarean does not refer to the way the Roman Emperor Julius Caesar was born, as some believe. It's actually taken from a Latin word, caedere, meaning 'to cut'.

EXPECTANT DADS' EXPERIENCES

Caesarean Birth

'We had to switch from a natural birth to a planned caesarean because the baby had turned at the last minute. Actually this may have been a blessing. The hospital will try and do everything they can to dissuade you from having a caesarean, and will give you lots of reasons for this. Having researched this quite a lot myself, I'm fairly strongly of the belief that they are primarily concerned at the cost – don't let the hospital staff influence you on this.'

Dominic N

The removal of the placenta

Whether your partner has a caesarean or usual – vaginal – birth, the third stage of labour will be the same: the removal of the placenta, or afterbirth.

Be warned, if the drama of the birth has left y
scarred for life, this final act could tip you over the ed
partner will have more contractions – even after your ch
been born – that will push the placenta out, but don't hold y
breath on this happening straight away. It can take up to an
hour. It's possible for your partner to have an injection of a drug
– Syntometrine or Syntocinon – that can speed this process up.
She would need to discuss this with the midwife before the birth
and specify it on the birth plan. It does mean that the placenta
is delivered within minutes of the birth.

You'll also need to alert the midwife if you intend to keep the
placenta. Some parents take it home, freeze it, then defrost it at
a later date and make it into a soup that mothers drink because
it's said to enrich the breastfeeding milk. In some cultures
parents bury the afterbirth – sometimes with books – in order
to ensure the baby grows up to be intelligent. Premier League
footballers covet its healing properties. Most of us leave it
behind for the hospital to do with as they please. Certainly don't
have it hanging around in the background when you're taking
your first baby pictures.

WILL I BE ABLE TO CUT THE CORD?

Cutting the cord has become something of a rite of passage
among many new dads these days. You may want to follow suit
– perhaps seeing it as a symbolic severing-of-the-ribbon occasion
opening the way to a new life for you all. Well, that's the flowery
version at least. In reality it's a messy moment that's over in a
flash – thankfully. If you are permitted to do it – hospital policy
or the obstetrician's call on the day could prevent you from
doing so – then one of the birth team will clamp the cord and
hand you a pair of surgical snippers. The cord links your baby to
its placenta – still inside your partner – on which it relied for
food and oxygen when it was in the womb. It contains one vein

and two arteries – the vein provided the nutrients and air, the arteries washed away its waste – and it measures about two centimetres in diameter. It's jellylike, covered in blood and fluid, about 60 centimetres long and the arteries are wound around the vein. As a result it's a bit of a bugger to cut through.

You're dealing with something akin to a greasy ship's rope at a time when all around you – partner, medical team, baby – seem to be screaming for you to get a bloody move on and do it.

In reality you and your partner should have a moment immediately after your baby is born to hold him or her as they're rested on the mother's chest. You'll then be able to cut the cord, though a few moments later it will be cut again by the delivery doctor about one centimetre away from the belly button. What's left of the cord on your baby's belly – a little stump – is disinfected and covered with a sterile bandage. About a week to 10 days after the birth the remnants of the cord will fall off – revealing your baby's belly button. The cutting of the cord doesn't hurt your baby, no matter how cack-handed you are.

Why should we store the cord stem cells?

In the past the umbilical cord would be cast away in the great mass of medical waste that some poor sod has to put out for the bin men on the Thursday morning – but now parents can opt to put the cord to life-saving use.

Part of the reason why the cord is such a tough nut to cut is because it's packed with your baby's stem cells. These cells can be extracted from the cord, stored and grown to become blood, bone or skin cells that can be used to repair damaged or diseased organs at any point in the next 20 years of your child's life.

By storing some of the blood and tissue from your baby's umbilical cord you will have a perfect match for their cells and blood. Right now, stem cells can be used to treat various cancers – such as leukaemia – and to provide an alternative to treatments such as bone marrow transplants, without the risk of

rejection or infection. In the future they may be
treat diabetes, heart disease and Parkinson's.

How are cord stem cells to be stored?

Here's the tricky bit. It's not something you can do yourself as a
keen new dad armed with just a penknife and Tupperware tub.

It's a task that has to be carried out by a doctor, midwife,
nurse or – here's another new pregnancy word – a phlebotomist,
qualified according to the Human Tissue Authority (HTA). At
present, out of the half a million-plus births in the UK every
year, only around a thousand stem cell samples are taken from
umbilical cords and banked.

It's not a common practice at all, but if it's something you
and your partner are interested in then ask your midwife or GP
at the earliest opportunity. You need to find out if your local
hospital trust has a licence to perform the process – different
trusts and different maternity units have varying policies when
it comes to stem cell storage.

Even then you may need to appoint a third-party specialist
to be on standby to remove and store the cells – there's also no
guarantee the cells can definitely be kept. There could be
complications surrounding the birth or the blood supply to your
baby that mean it's just not feasible to do it.

Of the stem cells that are saved at the request of parents,
the majority of them will be done where the baby is born in a
private, not NHS, hospital. This shouldn't deter you from
looking into the possibility of doing it, since the rewards for
storing something that will literally be thrown down a waste
chute otherwise are, quite literally, life-saving.

But don't pin your hopes on being able to go down this
route, and remember it comes at a cost too.

To find out more about stem cell storage speak to your GP
and midwife and investigate the advice offered by the Royal
College of Obstetricians and Gynaecologists, the Human Tissue

Authority and the Royal College of Midwives. Also take a look at the literature produced by such groups as Virgin Health Bank, who provide an accredited storage service. Their contact details are in the glossary.

CAN I TAKE THE PICTURE NOW OUR BABY IS BORN?

The first pictures you take of your newborn baby and, at this stage worn-out, partner may be kept for your own private perusal in a family album. Though, as is more likely the case, they'll be broadcast around the globe so that anyone who's ever known you can view them. At the very least you may have one framed to take pride of place on the mantelpiece for years to come.

It's best then if you let your partner have a few moments to compose herself, even do her hair or make-up (where's the overnight bag!). Be sure to let her finish breastfeeding before you dive in like a demented paparazzo taking shots of her. Turn off the flash too – the last thing your already startled baby needs is that thing going off.

Take a moment at this point to have a good long look at your child for the first time. And don't be too alarmed by what you see. Many newborn babies have the following – temporary – features.

Did you know?

Babies aren't Born Blind . . .

Babies can see when they're born – in fact if you shone a torch at your partner's abdomen before it was born your baby inside would blink. Don't do this though. It's not clever, for one thing, and it'll also add to any feeling of being a bit of a 'freak show' that your partner may have right now.

WHY DOES OUR BABY LOOK SO ODD?

At the moment of birth your baby will be a mix of red (oxygenated) and blue (de-oxygenated) blood. It'll most likely be covered in a white, waxy covering of vernix. The top of its head may be slightly bulging thanks to the suction effect of a ventouse if one was used, or else the sides of its head may have red imprints where the forceps were pressing against it. The umbilical cord will be blue, his or her lips and tongue will be a pinkish purple. All babies are born soaking wet, which is very handy. On meeting the cooler atmosphere of the outside world its skin cools, and this will trigger two reflexes – crying (the cold crying reflex – wet nappies have the same effect) and a rise in its blood pressure (the cold pressor reflex). So that it can cry, the baby needs to take a sharp deep breath – its first ever gasp of air! The combination of these reflexes will introduce your baby to breathing without the aid of the placenta.

WHY DO I FEEL SO ... UNDERWHELMED?

Some dads report feeling 'elated', 'overjoyed' or 'amazed' at the birth of their child. Pub-bore dads can drone on for days and in gory and gushing detail about the moment they saw their nipper for the first time. But don't fear that you're in some way odd if you're not doing cartwheels around the ward. Often the sheer trauma of the whole event can leave you stunned to the point where when you're finally holding your baby for the first time you struggle to say anything or know how to react. Your emotions will be all over the place with a sense of relief that the birth is over, concern about the health of your partner and just understandable ignorance as to what to do now.

Hold your baby!

That's what you should do now. If possible get one of the hospital staff to take a picture of you and your first baby. It's genuinely a moment in time you'll never relive exactly again and because we men, as fathers-to-be, often question our ability to live up to the task throughout the pregnancy it's a moment that takes on quite a bit of significance. Actually being able to hold a baby, your baby, in your arms for the very first time – you've done it. Allow yourself a little smug grin here, sunshine. Then prepare to . . .

Strip off!

Midwives and child experts agree that it's crucial for parents to hold their baby at this time as much as they can. So long as all is well with your little boy or girl you should seize the opportunity to do 'skin to skin' contact as soon as possible. According to studies carried out by Swedish researchers, a father having skin-to-skin contact with his newborn child will help calm them, especially if the mother is unable to hold the baby because she's just undergone a c-section. The same research also suggests that babies take to breastfeeding easier if they're first held by the dad then passed back to Mum – something to do with them nuzzling around your skin to find a milk supply, giving up hope, then experiencing great joy at latching on to your partner's breast. Something you can probably appreciate. So the upshot is, don't be afraid to whip off your shirt and hold your baby against your chest at the earliest opportunity – it'll stop you getting vernix all over your best Ben Sherman too.

EXPECTANT DADS' EXPERIENCES

Expect the Unexpected!

'We weren't ready for the moment when our baby's heart rate dropped or the vast list of statistics of possible problems the *anaesthetist gives you before giving the epidural or the amount of force used for a ventouse delivery, and the size of the suction cap they use. The fact there are lots of people there, and there are stirrups on the bed – it made sense, but I was a bit surprised to see it. The toughest thing was staying in hospital for five days for tests, and not knowing that there were 30 other babies, some critical, demanding doctors' attention, so we didn't get seen for two days.'*   Tom L

WHERE ARE THEY TAKING OUR BABY?

Within a few minutes of the birth the medical staff will perform a series of checks on your baby:

- **It'll be weighed.** Make a note of this. Once you start telling folk about the birth it's one of the first questions they'll fire back at you. You'll be told in pounds and kilos – jot down both as some smartarse relative who only works in metric will grill you on this.

- **It'll be measured.** The first of a long line of tests to see how tall your child is will begin now – it will develop into something of an obsession. Once you've taken your baby home your health visitor will give you a book in which to plot your child's growth. Then you'll buy a Height Chart for your kid's nursery – usually (and rather optimistically) with a giraffe on it. Then your kid's school will measure them when they're five years old . . . and so on.

- **It'll be tagged.** Hopefully this'll be the only time. The hospital will put an identity band on his or her wrist with the mother's surname on it. Don't fret, there's no need for you to tell the hospital the name of your baby right now.

- **It'll be tested.** A series of 'Apgar' tests are carried out several times on your baby after it's born. The midwife checks the **colour** of the baby's skin along with his or her **pulse, breathing, muscle movement** and **grimace** – the ability to pull a face or cry out as a reaction – and they are all then given a score. The highest Apgar score would be 10 (2 for each sign). The average, perfectly healthy child will usually score around 7. If a child scores between 4 and 6, some closer attention beyond routine postnatal care will be given to any low-scoring areas, though most babies who come in with a low score at first usually go on to be very healthy babies.

Some babies need extra help after their birth. If they were born premature or they have jaundice (see below) then the hospital will keep the baby and usually your partner in for observation and tests. If you know this is going to happen discuss with your partner how you want to play this before telling any others. Having an army of concerned relatives turning up outside the intensive care unit isn't going to help anyone. You don't have to lie. Just be a forceful new dad, insisting on no visitors unless you say otherwise. Lay down the law a little. It's good to get the practice for this in now.

CAN I TELL THE WORLD?

You're now a family. Share some family time together. You may be itching to tell the world the news but for now just take a moment to savour things. If you've got a present for your partner then now's the time to give it to her. Your partner may well be encouraged to breastfeed for the first time. She may find this a frustrating and uneasy experience. Provide the best support you can – even if this means leaving them be while you head off and make those calls you're dying to make. Prepare yourself as best you can by swotting up on answers for the questions you'll be hit with.

Telling friends and family the news

Tell one or two close relatives or friends your news then ask them to pass on the details. Tell them the essentials (below), then after the call switch off your phone for a while and go and have a lie-down.

- **Boy or girl?** In all the excitement, have you actually looked?
- **Weight?** Learn this in pounds, kilos and 'bags of sugar' (see below).
- **Time of birth?** People will want to know specifics – the exact time he or she appeared, how long your partner has been in labour for, Libran or Virgo, that kind of thing.
- **Distinguishing features?** Birthmarks, shock of ginger hair, 'he's hung just like his dad'. Give the gossip network something to chew over.
- **Who does he look like?** Any family members with blue-purple features, blood-matted hair, a ventouse-sucked crown and a white coating of vernix over their skin spring to mind?
- **Baby's name?** Unless you and your partner have positively, absolutely, implicitly decided on a name then don't reveal any of the possible ones right now. If people ask – and they will – say you're not sure yet and leave it at that. Don't let them try to and sway you or give out names that, thanks to Chinese whispers, you could become stuck with.

Quick Conversion Table for Baby Weights

The first question people ask about a new baby is 'boy or girl?' Then comes weight. Only women – mothers especially – know the true significance of a new baby's size and what it takes to catapult one into the world. If your brain's too scrambled to deal with decimal points or ounces, just tell them how many bags of sugar the baby weighed in at (1kg = 1 bag of sugar).

Metric	Old money	Sugar bags	Likely reaction from others
2.8kg	6lb 3oz	nearly 3	Good . . . not too big then
3.0kg	6lb 8oz	3	Good . . . healthy
3.3kg	7lb 4oz	more than 3	What's that, about average?
3.5kg	7lb 11oz	3½	Ooo . . . big 'un then?
3.8kg	8lb 6oz	nearly 4	Wahey! What a whopper!
4.0kg	8lb 13oz	4!	Ouch . . .

WHAT IS JAUNDICE?

Jaundice is a yellow taint to your baby's skin colouring that occurs because their liver is struggling to break down excess red blood cells. It's quite common and as long as baby is feeding well, alert and filling their nappy then this will soon fade. Depending on the severity of the jaundice the hospital may keep your baby in a special-care unit to sunbathe under an ultraviolet light that will help clear this up. In almost all cases babies born with jaundice go on to receive a completely clean bill of health.

DO I STAY WITH THEM OVERNIGHT?

Your partner may ask the medical team if you can be allowed to stay. Don't try to and get out of this by going off on one about 'hospital bugs' and how you 'need a decent night's sleep'. Instead, take the initiative and ask the midwife yourself. According to research from a government-backed Child Health Strategy there is 'strong evidence that early involvement of fathers has significant benefits for children's social, emotional and intellectual development and wellbeing'. To help get dads involved right from the off one of the key recommendations of the report is a call for strategic health authorities to support fathers staying overnight on maternity wards.

According to the National Childbirth Trust it can be quite a trauma for a father of a newborn baby to suddenly have to leave his partner and baby in hospital within hours of the birth, although sadly this is often what happens. Don't hold back in asking if there are facilities for you to stay at the hospital overnight if your partner and child have to. Some hospitals may be able to provide a space for you depending on how busy they are. Your partner will appreciate the support and you'll be on hand to share your child's first full morning in its new world. Just check on the parking meter though . . .

Bringing Home the Baby

Your Baby: Weeks 1–2

In the first week after your baby is born it will lose about 10 per cent of its body weight, caused mainly by fluid loss – urine and faeces including meconium, its first poo. Most newborns will be back to their fighting birth weight within about 10 days provided they're feeding well.

WHEN DO WE TAKE OUR BABY HOME?

When the midwife is happy that all is well with your baby (stuff is going in one end and coming out the other OK) and your partner can muster the energy to leave the bed then they'll be discharged. Paediatricians and midwives who have received specialist training will undertake an examination of a newborn before sending them home. This could happen within a few hours of the birth or maybe several days later if your baby has been kept in for observation or special treatment. If your baby has been born premature (earlier than 34 weeks) or underweight or needs extra help in breathing, feeding, generating body heat, or if they're suffering from any conditions affecting their heart or circulation the hospital will provide special care for them until the all-clear is given.

This can be a really tough time for both parents. You've just witnessed the birth of your little miracle and now you're not able to enjoy those touching first few moments that most fathers get to do.

The mass of clinical machinery in the special baby care units can add to your anxiety, though the staff working there are a very reassuring bunch. They'll usually encourage you to have as much contact with your baby as possible and will explain everything you need to know about handling your child at this time.

How do I get them home?

Once you have the all-clear you need to make your first journey as a new family. If you're driving them home from the hospital yourself you need to have a car seat for an age 0 child (see details in Chapter 5). This could be the car-seat-cum-carrier that comes with a travel system or a specific baby car seat.

Get familiar with fitting this before your baby is born to avoid spending hours wrestling with it on discharge day. If you're taking your baby home by taxi take your baby carrier along too. Taxi drivers, in the way they love to do, will tell you that the onus is on you – and not them – to make sure children are secure in the back of a taxi.

That very first night at home with your new baby isn't one you'll forget too soon. You probably won't sleep – despite being exhausted – and you'll undoubtedly stop to watch your infant sleep even though it will wake up every couple of hours. If your partner is breastfeeding – or even if she isn't – your kid's going to need some nourishment every couple of hours at least.

NEW DADS' EXPERIENCES

Bringing Home the Baby

'When we walked out of the hospital we felt that we were going to get stopped at any time and asked to take our baby back, as we didn't feel that we were qualified! We kept having to pinch *ourselves that we were parents and that we had to work out pretty quickly how to look after a new life. Mel had read a load of books before the birth, but it's not the same as having the baby there in real life. We got into it pretty quickly though and fortunately he wasn't too difficult a baby.'*   Matthew D

FEEDING

WHAT DO I DO WHEN SHE'S BREASTFEEDING?

As well as being the most natural method of giving your baby a decent dose of milk – along with immunity-boosting antibodies and essential growth nutrients – breastfeeding is also very cheap compared to the alternative. But, it's not as easy as it looks – and that's where you come in. New mums often experience problems getting their baby to connect their mouth on to their nipples to start feeding. If she doesn't crack this knack of getting your baby to latch on correctly it can cause problems for both mother and child. So for the first few feeds at least:

- Be there – and awake; you *can* help out.
- Encourage and comfort your partner as she perseveres with the breastfeeding – especially since it can be quite painful and frustrating at first as mother and baby get acquainted with the whole procedure. As every midwife will tell you, breastfeeding is linked to a whole host of well-documented health benefits for both mother and baby. Breastfed babies are less susceptible to infection, allergies and becoming overweight, while mothers who breastfeed develop a closer bond, prompt the release of 'feel-good' hormones such as serotonin, and may even reduce their risk of contracting certain types of cancer.
- Fetch pillows or her favoured feeding cushion to help support her or rest the baby on.

- If needed, change the nappy before she starts feeding.
- Nip to the kitchen to fetch your partner a big glass of water or snacks – breastfeeding can last for an hour or more and during that time she'll be pretty immobile.
- You can literally lend a hand to help your partner get your baby to latch on to her breast – especially useful if your partner has had twins.

Expectancy Explained

Things Even You Never Knew about Breasts . . .

Be prepared for a lot of frustration as she gets into the swing of things. Just because your partner's breasts may have grown or 'engorged' to a scale you'd never imagined during the pregnancy doesn't mean that she has a constant supply of the white stuff for your child. Nor does being female make her a natural breastfeeder.

In order for your partner to produce milk your baby has to feed – the sucking motion triggers the mother's pituitary gland to gear up the milk-production hormones. The more she feeds the more milk she creates.

Sore nipples become a serious issue, so keep your hands off for the time being. Babies can be quite voracious at first; 'little and often' is recommended for the feeding routine so that the milk supply is established. Don't be surprised if your partner's boobs become something of a drip seemingly supplying your kid 24/7. Your baby will also go through growth spurts – the first after around 10 days – which will send them on a feeding frenzy.

You may also find yourself in the chemist, among other paternity-leave chores, asking for nipple shields for your partner. These are soft silicone devices – shaped like little Mexican hats – that slip over the nipple and areola to help the baby latch on, protect sore nipples or calm a speedy flow of milk.

These are not to be confused with nipple pads, which your partner may put inside her bra if her breasts randomly leak milk.

Once she's churning the stuff out at almost industrial production rates then you may be able to help out by feeding your baby yourself. Breastfed babies feed pretty frequently – every two to three hours. She can try to express milk via a pump into a bottle (e.g. Avent ISIS pump and bottle, £22.49 from Argos), which means her breasts can have a well-earned break. You can do the graveyard feeding shift while she catches up on her sleep.

OK, put like that it may not sound such a great idea but the chance to feed and bond with your baby this way shouldn't be missed. And of course, the less attachment your child has to your partner's breasts, the sooner you may be able to rekindle your own relationship with them. However, some new dads find the sight of their partner's mammaries serving the purpose that nature intended quite off-putting. Research shows that many men experience a drop in their libido and sexual desire when their partner has a baby. This is believed to stem from an evolutionary response to ensure the randy male doesn't stray when his cave woman needs him most – while also preventing him from pestering her for sex while her body is still recovering from the birth.

HOW DO I DO THE BABY FEEDS?

If you're going to take a turn feeding your baby (breast or formula) milk here's how it's done:

Check it's clean

Baby bottles and the teats (rubber caps) need to be sterilised. Steriliser kits come in several guises – get familiar with yours.

- Chemical: These use sterilising tablets or liquids. You make up the solution, then leave the bottles and teats to soak for 30 minutes. Rinse the bottles before filling with the baby-grow juice and make a fresh sterilising solution every day.
- Steam: Works like a kettle. Cleans the bottles in up to 15 minutes depending on how many you're sterilising. Let the bottles cool before using them.
- Microwave: The easiest without a doubt. Put the bottles and teats in a plastic tub along with some water. Press go (you know this bit, don't you?). Takes around six to eight minutes to steam-clean the bottles. Be sure to take care when opening the bottles to avoid getting a faceful of hot steam.

Follow the formula instructions

This isn't a new mobile phone you're dealing with here, so don't try to bluff it or find out as you go. If you're using formula you must follow the serving directions on the label. This will tell you how much to use according to your baby's age. Don't feel the urge to 'add a spoonful for luck' – stick to the recommended amount, which is usually one scoop of formula to one of cool, pre-boiled water – be sure to check!

Test the temperature!

Before you start, drip a little milk on to your wrist to see that it's not too hot. Breastfed babies will be used to warm milk so if you're taking stored milk from the fridge sit it in a jug of hot water for a few moments to warm it up a little.

Avoid the microwave

OK, it's easy and lots of parents do it, but using a microwave to warm up feeds carries the risk of you overheating the milk and seriously annoying your baby as you scald their mouth. There's also some debate as to whether you nuke precious nutrients by microwaving the formula. If you must do it, be sure to stagger the process by heating it for 10 seconds, then stopping and stirring it. Heat again for 10 seconds then stir it again. In total only heat it for 30 seconds and be sure to mix the solution vigorously before offering it to your baby.

Get comfy

Like an elderly relative on Christmas Day, some babies like to take a taster, then have a little nap, then wake up a few minutes later with one hell of a thirst. Find yourself a seat and hold your baby cradled in your arm with its head on your shoulder. Remember, once they're feeding it'll be tricky to move so prepare for the long haul – if you're in front of the TV keep the remote handy.

Fill the teat

Tilt the bottle so that the teat is kept full of milk. If your baby starts sucking in air because you're not holding the bottle right it'll get wind. Wind won't harm it but it'll give little junior the gripes and you'll get earache as he tells you how uncomfortable he is.

Do the wind thing

To 'wind' them simply rub their back while they're sat upright on your lap. Prepare for a burp or a mouthful of partially digested milk all over your trousers. To protect your clothes and so avoid this, grab a 'muslin' cloth from the large mountain of them you should have around the house at this time.

Talk to them

If you've already been talking to your partner's bump or reading to your baby while it was still in the womb (don't laugh, some dads do) then they will already recognise your voice. Use feeding time to talk some more and watch how your baby reacts – see if you can be the first out of you and your partner to raise a smile or a giggle from them. If they frown, they're usually pooing.

Do the bottling up

Don't just leave your empties lying around the house. Babies on a bottle-feed frenzy will go through at least a six-pack of milk or formula a day. Buy a bottle and steriliser set that takes six to eight bottles and be sure to keep plenty in supply.

NEW DADS' EXPERIENCES

Breastfeeding

'The first few days after the birth were really tough as Max had jaundice, and we thought he was sleeping well, but later found out that we should have been waking up and feeding him. He was also struggling to feed as his nose was blocked, and we found out that a couple of saline drops from the chemist acted like a miracle cure. You can never know enough – we read books and tried to start a routine of some sort, though it is not really possible at first. The best advice came from a midwife who said

*to us, "Do whatever it takes to get through the first six weeks".
Breastfeeding was really tough until we discovered nipple shields
existed – brilliant – and my wife used them for four to five weeks
before he could drink normally from the breast.'*   Tom L

WHAT IF MY PARTNER DECIDES NOT TO BREASTFEED?

Breast is best, there's no doubt about it. The milk is cheap and
nutritious. The act of feeding creates a bond between baby and
mother. Some studies suggest it can reduce the risk of breast
cancer in mothers. Breastfed babies are less likely to suffer with
allergies when older and there's also less chance of obesity
occurring in adulthood if you imbibe from the boob as a babe.
According to research from the University of Glasgow breastfed
babies have a reduced risk of growing into overweight adults.

Health professionals are zealous about it. But the truth – as
revealed by Department of Health studies – is that a fifth of
mothers who start breastfeeding stop within the first two weeks.
Another 36 per cent switch from breast to bottle within the next
six weeks. The World Health Organization recommends that
women breastfeed for at least the first six months of their baby's
life. But research carried out by groups such as the Information
Centre for Health and Social Care suggest that as few as 1 per
cent of new mums will still be breastfeeding at that point.

For many mums it can become too painful or burdensome to
persist with. Others, fearful of the 'sagging' effect a feeding baby
will have upon their figure, opt for the bottle as soon as possible.
Some just can't produce enough milk to keep the little guzzler
going. Whatever your partner chooses, support her as much as
you can. The midwife will tell you, as Melvyn Dunstall has told
me, that you should encourage her – for both their sakes – to
persist with breastfeeding and provide as much support as
possible.

HOW DO I DEAL WITH THE EMBARRASSMENT?

Some new dads can't wait for the moment to arrive when their partner switches from breast to bottle for good. They admit to feeling jealous that this newcomer is monopolising their partner's mammaries, or else the discomfort they feel when their partner whips out a breast in public to meet the demands of a ravenous nipper is too much to handle.

Consider the fact that your partner won't be feeling too cocksure about this either. As natural as it is, no woman – even topless models – will feel 100 per cent at ease trying to do as Mother Nature intended in a corner of Starbucks on a busy Saturday morning. What she'll most likely appreciate is her partner – you, the new father – stepping in and helping her out. Try:

- Getting a little closer to her and shielding her if she wants you to instead of feigning a sudden interest in Fair Trade coffee posters.

- Grabbing one of those muslin cloths you've been mystified by since you bought them to drape over her shoulder or help wipe up any mess if she wants it.

- Not getting too concerned about the reactions of others. Instead dwell on the fact that US research shows how the odours given off by breastfeeding have been shown to heighten sexual desire in childless women. This is totally pointless information, I know – but it takes your mind off the whingers who think breastfeeding 'shouldn't be allowed'.

What does breast milk taste like?

It doesn't come in Slush Puppy-like flavours – but the make-up of it will be affected by what your partner eats and how much liquid she drinks. Generally those new dads who do taste breast milk (three in every five according to one study) report that it has a 'sweet tang' and a 'watery consistency' with just a 'hint of vanilla'.

When your child feeds it gets a thirst-quenching foremilk, followed by the more calorific, nutritious hindmilk. But in the first three to four days your partner's breasts produce a much stronger solution altogether – a substance called colostrum. She may have been leaking a little of this for the past few weeks already. This 'Full Cream' of the breast-milk range is revered for its laxative effect – it'll bring on your kid's first poo.

NAPPIES

This first poo will be nine months' worth of backed-up waste. It's such a poo that it even comes with its own name: the meconium. It's usually black, sticky and resembles the stuff Greenpeace have to wash off seagulls. It looks worse than it smells – sadly that isn't the case with all that follows.

IS BABY POO AS BAD AS EVERYONE SAYS?

Yes. Also your baby's poo will dominate the conversations you and your partner have for months to come. Lines like 'He did a real stinker today!' or 'I really drew the short straw with this nappy change!' will enter common parlance and replace the everyday little chats you and she used to have about hangovers, what's for dinner or the like. After the meconium, the texture, shade and nasal 'tones' you get from their poo changes:

- They can be loose, orange/yellow inoffensive ones, which are more common in breastfed babies.
- Or the eye-watering, solid, brown type, often deposited by babies drinking formula milk.

- Occasionally, when a baby is changing from breast to bottle, its poo can take on a green hue, though this can also occur in babies suffering with colic (see 'Crying' below).

Perhaps the most surprising element is the amount of poo your little 'un can produce. Every baby is different in the quantity and consistency they deliver, though the fact they they're using all the milk they take (particularly if they're being breast-fed) to function and grow means they can go for a few days without pooing – only to save one up especially for your shift. Equally, some can go three or four times a day!

If you watch closely you'll notice how your child's facial features will change – often frowning or seemingly deep in thought – when they poo. This isn't a proven fact, but I bet when your kid does that you'll find it's doing one.

WHAT ABOUT THE WEE?

Much like the similar-sounding Wii, you could find yourself enjoying a little home entertainment with your baby's pee – especially if you have a boy.

Even at a few days old they're capable of sending spiralling jets of urine over great distances like the water cannon used by continental riot police. This usually occurs at the exact moment you remove their nappy – when the air temperature around their bladder changes, triggering the hose effect. Thankfully this jet wash isn't as odorous as the adult variety.

There's no rule as to how often your baby will need their nappy changed – a ballpark average is six a day – but they should certainly wee a few times a day. If they're suffering with diarrhoea or peeing profusely then you need to talk to your baby's GP or the health visitor.

HOW DO I CHANGE THE NAPPY?

Once you're decided on which nappies you're using then the method of changing them will follow one of two routes.

Reuseable nappies

These are said to be more eco-friendly. However, one report by the Department for Environment, Food and Rural Affairs found that the terry type – with the additional washing required – actually have a higher carbon footprint than their disposable equivalents, although reuseable nappies can be chucked in with a normal load.

However, the landfill effect of the throwaway variety isn't much better – notice how your refuse sack quota doubles when you start using disposable nappies.

Reuseable nappies also require a number of accessories such as nappy pins, liners, plastic pants – although these are one-off costs.

In the past there was an element of origami to putting a reuseable nappy on a baby – including such moves as the 'newborn fold', 'T fold' and 'kite fold'. Diagram instructions are provided and there's even YouTube stuff on this. Today, however, reuseable ones have become as easy to fit as disposables.

Disposable nappies

Many parents instead opt for the disposable type – they're costlier but more convenient.

To change either, follow a few simple rules.

- Do it on the floor – on a changing mat. That way you don't risk your kid wriggling out of your reach.
- Get all the extras – wipes, cream, biodegradable disposal bags and fresh nappy – ready beforehand.

- Undo nappy-fastening, gag (especially if they're drinking formula milk, which seems to make their poo smell worse) and remove nappy. As you change more nappies and become more accomplished – OK, *if* you change more and become more accomplished – you'll find you're able to wipe some of the excess poo from your baby's bum using the clean part of the nappy, then fasten it all into a bundle. It also saves on using up wipes and nappy bags. Wipes cost about 0.01p but this remains an early fathering skill that some seem particularly proud of.

- Dispose of the old one (just fold and seal or place in the scented bags for disposables or the bucket with a lid on for reuseable ones). Wipe your baby's bum using wipes or cotton wool and warm water. Dry them thoroughly then apply barrier cream if you're using it.

- Slide the clean nappy under your baby, bring the front up through (between) the legs and fasten with the tabs at the side.

- Dress your baby then wash your hands. Sniff your hands. Wash them again.

Did you know?

Nappy Washing Services

Washing nappies is a grim, almost constant job. The average baby will get through 5,000 nappies before it's finally potty trained. Mindful of this, enterprising types following that old adage about 'where there's muck there's brass' have set up nappy washing services. For around £9 a week you can have your reuseables collected, cleaned and returned to your door. It's a weekly service so you'll need to keep the used ones in a deodorised bucket with a lid between collections – to find your nearest service visit the National Association of Nappy Services (NANS) at www.changeanappy.co.uk/information.htm.

Did you know?

Cloth Cuts

Terry nappies first appeared in the late 19th century when changes in fabric weaving methods led to the mass production of the absorbent cloth. Prior to that cotton cloths and rags were used. The first disposable nappies were developed in Sweden in the 1940s and featured throwaway tissues worn inside rubber pants.

HOW DO I BATHE OUR BABY?

Bathing your baby could actually soothe and relax you too. While mothers and babies are believed to 'bond' through the chemical exchange of oxytocin – a hormone passed through breast milk – it's believed that the warm soothing experience of bathing a baby provokes the release of oxytocin in dads. It works for your kid because it's oxytocin that helps humans remember strange faces. It's a hormone that's also produced during lovemaking and so is believed to play a part in helping couples to bond as well (therefore lovemaking in the bath could seal man and woman for life). Anyway, back to the point, bathtime won't just chill the pair of you out and help you get closer. Studies carried out at the University of Central London found that children were three times more likely to experience behavioural problems later in life if they were not bathed regularly by both parents as youngsters. When it's Dad's turn to bathe baby remember the basics.

- Check the water isn't too hot – that traditional image of Dad dipping his elbow in the bath isn't far removed from fact. Unlike your hands, which may be used to hot water (or were before you bought the dishwasher), your elbow is more sensitive to hot or cold. The water for your baby should be tepid/warm for your elbow.

- Have all the gear – cloths, baby shampoo, towel, rubber ducky etc. – nearby. Never leave your nipper alone to swim freestyle in the bath, not even for a few moments.

- Support them with one hand and gently swish the water over them with the other. If you're using soap avoid putting it over your baby's face.

- Make funny faces and noises to relax your child (hopefully). Even though they spent nine months paddling in an amniotic sac they still find baths a bit bemusing on the whole.

- Dab them dry with a towel. Apply whatever lotions and potions your partner's invested shares in. Dress them just in time for them to poo or spew again.

VISITORS

WHAT'S THE BEST WAY TO DEAL WITH THE CROWDS OF VISITORS?

Among the many new roles you're taking on at this point there's also that of gatekeeper. Often a newborn and mum are subjected to lots of visits by friends and family. The advice of midwives is to let them visit, of course, but try to limit the time people stay for. Also make sure visits are spaced out, as for an exhausted new couple there can be nothing worse than a houseful of baby admirers.

Visitors do love saying things like 'Is there anything you need? Anything? Just ask . . .' Take them up on such offers. Ironing, making meals, taking baby for a walk around the block in the buggy, more ironing – anything you don't want to do, be sure to make them feel they're helping out by picking up the slack.

If there's a sibling or stepbrothers or -sisters encourage visitors to include siblings too, as the new baby will be the centre of attention and some brothers or sisters find it difficult to deal with. Sometimes these early signs of preferential treatment can nurture feelings of resentment that make for gruesome family feuds in years to come! Warning enough?

Perhaps the greatest help, or hindrance, at this point will come from the wise old matriarchs in your family. Plenty of new mums find the support and advice of their own mothers or even their mother-in-law comes in handy at this time. You, however, may not find the intrusion into the life of YOUR new family so easy to deal with. Sometimes it's the mother-in-law's dominance of things, using terms like 'it was good enough in my day' when rubbing goose fat into your baby's chest, or it may just be that they always seem to be around the house or holding your baby when you want to.

If you're having problems dealing with it begin by talking it through with your partner – it could be that she's thinking the same but doesn't want to say anything for fear of causing offence or losing the support of the mother-in-law completely. Don't put pressure on your partner to say something if she's not in agreement with you – she'll have enough on her plate right now.

Instead reach some kind of agreement on just how much help you want from your relatives and when you want it. Make sure they know that you genuinely appreciate their support but that you feel it's now time for you and your partner to start learning how to fend for yourselves as parents. Keep it tactful, possibly set specific days or times when visits should take place or, if for instance your mother-in-law's staying with you, discuss how you want things to be when you return from work and want to spend time with your partner and baby.

Most of all be unified with what your partner wants and what you both feel is best for your baby. Any squabbles you have now with the in-laws will heal in time and any ground rules you lay down now will help when you have your next child . . . In the meantime other ways of dealing with the influx of well-wishers include:

Switch on the answerphone

Leave a brief message about the birth and how mother and baby are well then let folks leave messages. Call them back when you're up to it.

Put mobiles on silent

Yours – and get any guests to as well. To have an almost-napping baby suddenly shocked back into wailing mode by the Nokia chimes can infuriate an already fraught new mother.

Set times

The baby will get into a feeding routine, so if you're going to have guests it may be worth trying to time any visits around this or nap time. When friends say, 'When can we come and see the little 'un?' then check in with the breast diary first.

Have a code

Create a code word that you and your partner can use during visits. If any guests are outstaying their welcome then she can use the code word and you can initiate an evacuation by scooping up the tea and biscuits and ushering guests to the door.

NEW DADS' EXPERIENCES

Crowd Control

'Do NOT invite anyone round to see the baby for at least a week. Your wife either gets paranoid about exposing the baby to germs

or feels uncomfortable because the house is a tip and she looks like crap. Also it's too stimulating for the baby – so they scream either during or after and then won't settle. I ended up serving tea and biscuits when we should both just have been relaxing and getting to know our baby. If there's anyone you really want to see – go and visit them, then you can leave when you're ready (we had some people staying for hours!). Or meet people for a stroll in the park with the baby in the pram.' Paul S

CAN WE TAKE OUR BABY OUTSIDE BEFORE IT'S BEEN VACCINATED?

You can indeed. Once you've mastered the basics regarding what goes in to your baby and how to deal with what comes out then the rest of the time is your new 'family' time – with the exception of sleeping and crying and having to go back to work and arguing . . . which we'll come to.

Taking your baby out to see their new world will be an anxious moment. The first trip beyond the front door as a family will get you used to the fact that you can no longer just grab your door keys, wallet and phone and go. From now on any excursion involving you and the baby will take on the kind of logistics you associate with major military exercises – especially since you'll overpack the buggy. 'Just in case we need it . . .' will become your family motto.

While you're out, buy a baby carrier if you haven't already. These papoose-like harnesses have become a badge of virility among modern dads. Wearing one allows you to announce to the viewing public, 'I made this kid, I'm a caring dad – come and take a look, especially cooing females.' They're available in a range of designs and colours including sleek black ones and shades that'll match your favourite football team shirt. A few things to consider when buying and first using one are:

- Head support. Although the harnesses can be used from very early on, most babies are – structurally – little more than a bag of over 300 bones. They're unable to hold up their own heads until they're about four months old when their muscles start to form and bones fuse together. Ensure you've got a carrier that supports them fully and to begin with you'll carry them so that they're facing you – so that their head is comfortably propped up between the harness's support and your chest.

- Try before you buy. As with fold-down buggies, there's a knack. Most harnesses, like the BabyBjörn range of traditional-style carriers, are Velcro-and-strap arrangements. Get used to fitting it securely to you at first then securing the fastenings before you put your baby in.

- Test drive your baby carrier. Walk around indoors, try out the stairs, negotiate bends, get familiar with the effect it has on your balance. Do sitting down and taking the blasted thing off again. Try all with baby *in situ* before leaving the house.

- Don't suffer the slings. Baby carriers – the harness type where they're strapped to your back or chest – wear well on a bloke. They provide a secure and sensitive bond between you and your baby. Slings are a different deal altogether. These are recumbent earth-mother bags that hold the baby at the side, the same way you may have done with a sack of Sunday broadsheets on a paper round. They have their place, but it's not on a man.

- Grab a dad bag. Camouflage? Retro style? Sporting backpack or LP carrier design? Baby-gear marketers have wised up to the style requirements of the kid-conscious new-age dad. Now you can get a stylish carry-all pack that'll hold less butch items – like baby wipes – beneath an all-action exterior. Mothers call these 'changing bags' and aren't so self-conscious.

Taking Baby Out – Proud Dad Essentials

Heading out into the big wide world with your brand-new baby? Be sure to take:

- The carrier/harness: if you're not taking the buggy then get the straps secure and baby in place before you leave the house.
- The dad bag: containing . . .
- Changing mat (optional).
- Baby wipes and disposal bag (obligatory).
- Nappies (downright essential).
- Baby formula/milk, bottles and bib (ditto).
- In the summer: sun hat and sun screen (at least SPF 50 or complete sunblock) for the baby, though most health visitors suggest you keep your baby out of direct exposure to the sun completely – especially since their skin will be very sensitive and could react badly to the sun cream.
- In the winter: woolly hat, additional blankets, extra layers for cold weather trips.
- The car seat: if you can't be bothered with carrying all of the above and would rather just take them for a drive.

REGISTERING THE BIRTH – WHY DO I HAVE TO GO ALONG?

As new parents one of your first duties will be to register your baby. You need to do this within six weeks – or 42 days to be precise – of the birth at your nearest Registry Office (listed in the phonebook or on your Local Authority website). If you're not married, the mother must register the birth – if she wants

the father's name to appear on the birth certific[a]
father must go along too.

If you're married then you can register the birth y[ou]
You need to tell them:

- The date and place of your child's birth
- The forename, middle name (plus others if you've named them after your all-time football XI) and surname that you've chosen for them
- The name, birth date, place of birth and occupation of the father
- The name, birth date, place of birth and occupation of the mother

In return you'll get: a Birth Certificate for your child, which in turn will open up a whole new world of red tape and bureaucracy to them. It'll also mean they can be registered with a GP, get access to any funds they're entitled to such as their child benefit, have written proof that 'You are the daddy' etc.

SLEEP

SHOULD WE LET OUR BABY SLEEP IN WITH US?

After shelling out for all that bedroom furniture you may feel a bit miffed if your partner suddenly suggests a threesome that involves your baby becoming a physical bolster between you both once more. On the other hand it can be quite a touching experience to share your bed with the little life the pair of you have created.

Although many parents admit to doing it, the experts advise against it due to the risk of accidental smothers. Of course, not all experts agree. The Royal College of Midwives say that bed-sharing encourages bonding and helps with breastfeeding.

Only do it if you both want to. It's not a great idea if you sleep on a waterbed and definitely a no-go if you've been drinking, are taking medication that makes you drowsy or are active smokers. Also, your own fear of performing a Big Daddy-style splashdown as a 15-stone father rolling over on to his newborn baby may stop you sleeping soundly anyway. Most importantly, don't make a habit of it.

Did you know?

Tot Pants

New babies at rest breathe between 40 and 50 times per minute. By age five it drops to around 25 times per minute.

HOW SHOULD I PUT OUR BABY TO SLEEP?

Sleep is one area likely to send new parents into tortuous paranoia. Because the exact cause of cot death or Sudden Infant Death Syndrome – which claims the lives of around 300 babies every year – isn't known, any midnight gurgling or radio silence from the baby-listening device can strike fear into the hearts of first-time parents.

The advice to follow – from the Foundation for the Study of Infant Death (FSID) and the Department of Health – when you're putting your baby to bed is to be sure to:

• Keep their room temperature between 16 and 20 degrees C (get a room thermometer) and don't have the cot next to a radiator.

- Lie them on their back. The FSID line is to make sure you place your baby with their feet to the foot of the cot – this stops them from wriggling down under their covers – though using a baby sleeping bag should prevent this too.

- The experts also maintain that the safest place for your baby to sleep is in a crib or cot in a room with you for the first six months.

- Feel your baby's chest. If they feel warm to you, then they're probably warm enough. If they're hot or sweaty, remove some of the layers. If they're cold, add more layers to warm them.

- If they seem unwell, hot and shivery, remove a few layers so that they cool down.

- Avoid putting teddies in the cot – and definitely don't smoke in your child's room, and ideally not even in the house from now on.

Did you know?

Squeals on Wheels

One in four parents surveyed by kids' car seat firm Graco claimed to have driven their babies on average up to 30 miles a week in the car to settle them to sleep. Some parents had even resorted to leaving electrical items, ranging from hairdryers to Hoovers, switched on and running in an attempt to use the 'white noise' created to settle their inconsolable infants.

For many new dads the image of you lying there on the sofa channel-hopping while your newborn lies snugly snoozing on your chest is a magical moment you may have been secretly aspiring to. Certainly, if your baby wants to take a nap on your chest during the day while you're fully awake it's no bad thing – a great photo opportunity in fact (as if your partner didn't already have enough to do without having to take snaps of the proud dad).

However, this picture of serenity doesn't come without a warning. The FSID advice on sharing a bed with your baby is pretty clear and when it comes to sharing a bed with your baby when you've been drinking or taking drugs it's downright adamant. Basically, don't do it! Now it seems the same should be said of sharing a sofa with your sleeping baby too. A report published through the *British Medical Journal*'s website claims that half of all cot deaths were linked to the baby sleeping with Mum or Dad – and a 'high proportion' of these occurred when the parent and baby fell asleep on the sofa. To avoid the unthinkable, take care when feeding or relaxing with your baby on the sofa. If you're tired or have been drinking ask your partner to take over this time. They can do the feed or put your baby down in their cot or crib while you take to the couch or bed on your own. Don't use this as get-out policy, though – she'll soon twig.

Did you know?

Don't Sleep Like a Baby

Newborn babies sleep between 14 and 18 hours a day. But not all in one block. A constant appetite and much shorter sleep cycle than us – in which they spend most of their time in 'light' REM sleep – is why a sleeping baby is only ever one heavy-footed clump on the floor away from waking and wailing like a car alarm.

NEW DADS' EXPERIENCES

First Weeks

'When we got home it did feel strange to have this other little person there. My wife said it felt odd knowing that she would never be able to 100 per cent relax because she'd always be wondering if she was sleeping/needed feeding/changing etc. You do both get a bit paranoid. Our baby monitor was set so loud we could hear her breathing (a mistake, I think) so that if for some reason her breathing became quiet (which it does, obviously) we'd panic!'

Paul S

CRYING

HOW DO I STOP OUR BABY FROM CRYING?

Some babies cry incessantly, others you'll hardly hear a peep out of. (The latter ones are a myth created by parents trying to erase the hell from their memories.) The first week may be peace and tranquillity. Newborns spend most of the first fortnight dozing. It can be a bit of an anticlimax for the excited new dad on paternity leave. However, by the third week they could be in what seems like 24/7 tearful meltdown. With serious effects. Recent research from the Netherlands suggests that crying babies not only put their parents' love to the test, but also strain their mum and dad's sanity – to the point that crying is believed to be a major cause of postnatal depression in mothers and fathers.

The reasons why your baby cries will vary. Once you're familiar with their patterns then the obvious can be ticked off – feed, wet nappy, needs a nap etc. For both mums and dads holding a crying baby can be a demoralising act. You feel you're not doing things right. A common cause of near-constant crying is colic. This can start at around two weeks and reach a peak after about six weeks.

It basically means crying a lot, though it sounds as if there should be a medical remedy. There isn't, though that doesn't stop people from marketing supposed colic cures. Among the varied techniques that parents have employed to settle a baby who is not hungry or tired but has a bad case of the gripes are:

- **Taking turns:** Don't assume that she'll have any better technique in dealing with the tears than you will.

- **Shhh:** Comes naturally and involves a gentle 'shushing' noise or even singing while carrying your baby in your arms. If it works it's possibly because it re-creates the white noise your baby heard in the womb – it's more likely though that they're just stunned into silence by how bad your singing is.

- **Walking:** Just a change of scenery or room temperature can be enough to settle your child.

- **Whirring:** Not you. Machines. Among the various tactics employed by desperate dads include strapping the kid into the car and driving it to sleep, turning on the hair drier to harness that 'white noise' fetish babies have, and even putting a radio in the baby's room (not necessarily to any station – the 'white noise' provided by the interference between stations could do even better) might help. In fact a team from Queen Charlotte's Hospital in London found that 80 per cent of babies aged between two and seven days old fell asleep within five minutes in response to white noise – but just 25 per cent fell asleep without it in the same amount of time.

Your baby will grow out of colic – though it could be up to 12 weeks after they're born that they start settling down. The sound of your baby wailing again as you approach the front door on the way home from work can make even the most devoted dad want to turn on his heels. 'Stick it out' is the best advice here – evenings are often the worst time for colic-stricken babies, but it will get better.

Did you know?

Babies Don't Actually Cry . . .

That's right, they may be howling the house down but don't say your kid is crying because – technically – it's not. Newborns don't shed tears because their tear ducts haven't fully formed. But after about four weeks – once the ducts have had a chance to develop – they can weep tears. On the down side – for your nipper – they're unable to wash out their eyes the way we grown-ups do, so be aware that anything that gets in its eyes will cause it some discomfort for a while. Look out for it blinking a lot – you'll notice this because their reflex actions aren't developed either. As a result babies only blink, naturally, on average about four times a minute. (We blink 12 to 20 times every 60 seconds). Never get into a staring contest with your baby. You don't stand a chance . . .

NEW DADS' EXPERIENCES

Sleep Deprivation

'Because we were both party animals prior to the pregnancy we kind of thought we'd not be so concerned about the lack of sleep thing. But we were wrong. You just don't get a chance to catch up. I sat up with Michelle during the night feeds but by the second week of my paternity leave I started copping out – pretending to be asleep – when he woke every two hours. I feel guilty about it now still. Those are tough times but you get through them.'

Paul S

12

The Six-week MOT...

Your Baby: Weeks 3-6

Newborn babies are maligned for 'not doing much' in the first few weeks of life. Admittedly they're quite predictable – crying, feeding, pooing and sleeping – but there's more going on than meets the eye. Their memory is kicking in already – they'll recognise friendly faces and will mimic expressions you make. They can pile on another 3lb (1.4kg) in weight and several inches in height (well, length, since they're not standing up yet) by the end of the first six weeks.

Expectancy Explained

The Health Visitor

The emotional state of new parents will ebb and flow – from a state of paranoia about the health of their baby, to being elated, pinching themselves, or just out-and-out exhausted. If your baby does have any development problems or ailments you may not be able to tell – which is why you have a new busybody-cum-house-guest in the shape of your health visitor.

Your partner will receive regular drop-in home calls from the health visitor. The first of these will be a couple of days after the birth. They will check the baby's measurements, look for any signs of illness and, most importantly, provide you both with advice and answers to any questions. Aside from the more obvious problems – cuts, bruises or choking – other signs you should seek advice about include:

- Changes in skin colouration; looking pale, yellowing of the skin or rashes appearing.
- Fever, difficulty in breathing or shortness of breath.
- Being sick; i.e. actual vomiting as opposed to the occasional up-chuck of milk or formula.
- Drowsiness, feeling limp or floppy, or showing no interest in feeds.

Do speak up if there's anything that doesn't strike you as being 'right' about your baby. If the health visitor isn't around and you think there's something wrong then get straight on to your GP or NHS Direct (www.nhsdirect.nhs.uk).

After six weeks your partner will have a checkup with her GP or back at the hospital. These are designed to ensure there are no postnatal problems and include a blood pressure reading, checks on the healing of any stitches she may have had, urine tests and answers to any questions she may have.

WHICH PROBLEMS SHOULD WE TREAT OURSELVES?

Babies have the oddest ailments. Your health visitor or GP will give you the best advice on how to treat them. Most will clear up in time but some can be dealt with by a dexterous hands-on Dr Dad . . . Yes, that's you. Here's how:

Problem: Cradle cap

A cute name for a scabrous rash – mild eczema – forming on the scalp.
Solution: Rub olive oil over the scab, leave overnight then shampoo out.

Problem: Croup

A seal-like barking cough – honest!
Solution: It's caused by mucus in the throat, possibly linked to an infection. Run a hot tap in the bath and sit with them – in the bathroom, not the bath itself – as they breathe in the steam and so ease the cough.

Problem: Sticky eye

Discharge from the tear ducts causes eyelids to stick together.
Solution: Gently clear each eye with a separate dab of cotton wool soaked in (boiled-then-cooled) water. Breast milk has also been found to be a natural means of clearing it up. You may want to ask your partner to perform that trick.

HOW DO WE KNOW IF THEY'RE DEVELOPING OK?

It's a little early to be singling junior out for a scholarship but there's no harm in doing a few development checks – if nothing else they will liven up your time spent holding them.

- Get grasping. Check out their ability to provide a strong handshake by placing your little finger in the palm of their hand to test their reaction and grip. Limp? Firm? Freemason?

- Tickle toes. After about four weeks your baby's movement will have developed to a point where they will bend their leg at the knee or retract their foot if you tickle the sole. Try it! It's great fun and certainly something you couldn't do with a pet dog.

- Take steps. Your baby will make walking movements when you hold them upright but you have to make sure to support their head. Resist the urge to drag them backwards while calling out, 'Look, love, she can Moonwalk.'

- Use light. From the first few weeks your baby's focus will be drawn towards the window – not because they want to escape but because the light (and bright colours) will capture their attention. See if you can get them to follow you with their eyes – playing 'peek-a-boo'-style games when changing them.

- Talk up. By around the six-week point your baby will be smiling and may even begin responding to your speech by making noises too. Treasure these moments, when this 'back-chat' that they give you is devoid of any attitude . . . it doesn't last.

WHY THE EMPHASIS ON GETTING OUR BABY INTO A ROUTINE?

We are all, as they say, creatures of habit, and those habits begin early on in life. Just after the birth, in fact, as parents soon learn the beauty of establishing a routine for their babies. At first they sleep and eat in a fairly random way but over the space of a few months you and your partner will learn how to stop your baby crying when they're hungry or overtired by nurturing a routine.

You learn from their pattern of demands and soon establish a structure to the times they feed, they sleep, they feed again, they need a change, they have a bath, they go down for the night (hopefully). Establishing a routine not only saves your sanity and allows you some structure to your life but it acts as a useful warning tool.

Once you have a routine in place then you'll find it easier to spot something is wrong – they're suddenly crying when they're neither tired nor hungry, for example. (Although they do go through growth spurts that mean you have to readdress the routine at various times.) This all may sound pretty simple but it's an incredibly useful thing to observe and learn – especially since your baby has no other means of communicating with you at this time. Once the routine is established, do your utmost to avoid breaking it.

NEW DADS' EXPERIENCES

Getting into Routines

'I would recommend that you get your baby into a routine as early as possible. Bath her in the evening from week three, and then put her to bed. If you are like us, you will then find that she cries/wants to feed from about five till nine on average, but that gradually calms down. I would say that she got into a routine by about week 10, and is now sleeping through from seven till five-thirty. Also we found that the key to getting her to sleep is to make sure she feeds properly when she goes to bed – the best way of doing this is to feed her from a bottle (using expressed milk) at about 6 p.m. – make sure she drinks the lot, and if she doesn't, leave the bottle in the room as you will need it soon after when she wakes up.'

Dominic N

HOW CAN I HELP MY PARTNER GET OVER THE 'BABY BLUES'?

To begin with avoid using the words 'baby blues' – not around her, anyway. It is a bona fide term health professionals use when referring to a brief droop in a new mother's mood in the days immediately after the birth. Often it's the result of exhaustion, trauma, fluctuating hormones and a fair dose of anxiety about the baby. These 'blues' are not something GPs are likely to prescribe anything for, since in most cases they will ease within a few days – but some mums take exception to such cosy terminology being used to explain how they feel.

Also be on guard for signs of the more serious postnatal depression (PND) or postnatal psychosis. God forbid you simply brush this mother of all downers off with terms like 'baby blues'. This can be a devastating illness and it's not one we 'superdads' can fix or easily solve no matter how much we want to. Equally, hoping she'll 'snap out of it' isn't a sound approach either.

In the bulk of cases it's the new father who's the first to witness symptoms of depression in their partner. Your actions at this time could be pivotal in helping her deal with it and so ensure the health and wellbeing of your entire family. It's estimated that possibly four out of five new mums suffer with some form of PND. It can kick in almost immediately after the birth – in the form of the 'baby blues' – but then worsen. Alternatively, it can slowly overwhelm her, possibly several months down the line from the birth. Many mums find the period immediately after their husband's return to work an especially tough time.

HOW CAN I TELL IF SHE HAS PND?

This depression can take many forms: from sporadic mood swings that pass as quickly as they come, through to weeks, months and in some cases years filled with bouts of emotional anguish, tears and feelings of self-doubt.

If the thought 'run away' springs to mind at this point, you're not alone in thinking it. But almost as if Mother Nature knew you might react this way there's an evolutionary brake applied to new dads that is automatically applied after the birth to stop such scarpering. In the weeks immediately following the birth your testosterone levels can drop by around 30 per cent. Experts believe it's nature's way of making us less aggressive, less likely to take stupid risks now that we have responsibilities, and a sure-fire way of stopping us sodding off the minute the baby's born or the effects of the birth send our wives into temporary meltdown.

It doesn't stop all new dads from shirking their role, of course – but in almost all cases of PND, with the support of a considerate and supportive husband most new mothers come through it OK.

In more extreme cases – estimated to be around 10 per cent – the mother will need the help of her GP or a healthcare specialist. The effect of an illness like this isn't restricted to the woman suffering with it either. She may feel an indifference to the baby, a resentment to you and the 'freedom' you have compared to her new role at home with the newborn. The symptoms of PND to look out for can include:

- Feeling low, telling you she's feeling down (fairly obvious then that something's up) or a lack of interest in the baby.
- Tearfulness and heightened irritability (you annoy her more than usual). She might start making statements about 'coping' or not feeling up to the role of motherhood.
- Forgetfulness, poor appetite and loss of energy.

These are signs you *may* be able to see. Because women with PND are often fearful of being seen as inadequate or unable to cope as mothers, your partner may do her best to put on a brave face. You're going to have to make a point of sitting down with her as often as possible and getting her to talk to you about how she's feeling.

Ask how you can help out more around the home if she feels she needs you to.

Be there. Ease up on the after-work social whirl and poker nights for a few weeks at least. If she's feeling upset about her situation then she's going to feel doubly bad when you text to say you're not coming home until late after she's sat at home all day with only a three-week-old for conversation.

Arrange visits to friends, to the park, to the beach, anywhere that isn't the four walls of home. Her GP will most likely prescribe such activities as part of a recovery plan if she goes down the medical route, so get in there first by encouraging her to take a break from the baby for an hour or two and see a friend, or have a babysitter you trust come around.

The health visitor will ask your partner how she's coping but again the fear of being seen as a failure may prevent her from speaking up. You can play a starring role here by alerting the health visitor to any worries you have about your partner. You've got to tread carefully, as she may feel in an already fragile state and won't appreciate you going behind her back, but for her health, the love of your child and your sanity too don't be afraid to ask the visitor for help.

Don't think that you're being more of a hindrance than a help with this. Studies carried out in Canada found that where the husbands and partners of new mums suffering with PND actively supported their wives, the women displayed a decrease in depression symptoms. According to research published by the National Childcare Trust, fathers can act as a 'buffer' for the negative effects a mother's depression can have on their child too. But this can take its toll on you.

Did you know?

Baby Bells

A baby crying reaches a sound measure of around 110 decibels (db). That's not as loud as an ambulance siren (120db) but is louder than an electric drill (100db), heavy traffic (85db) and a ringing phone (80db).

Do dads *really* get postnatal depression?

They do, though the symptoms of depression in new fathers are different and the statistics suggest it's a lot less common. This condition, a phenomenon that is no doubt somewhere called 'the daddy blues', affects around one in every 25 new fathers in the UK. Research from Denmark – looking at the subject of depression in men – found that new dads were twice as likely to have the 'blues' as experienced fathers. The Danish researchers noted that many dads ticking the postnatal depression box exhibited the following symptoms:

- Feeling a lack of support or involvement from the mother
- Feeling that the quality of the couple's relationship was not strong in the first place
- Feeling that there were disagreements about the pregnancy and how to deal with problems with the baby

Whether we dads suffer with postnatal depression as such is open to debate, but there's no doubt the huge upheaval in lifestyle coupled with the added responsibility, the trauma of seeing your partner go through the birth, the sleepless nights, the added expense and the lack of sex or even attention from your other half can take its toll.

In those first few months you will feel tired, irritable, clueless at times and even regretful – along with jealous, sex-starved and resentful as you watch your kid monopolise your partner's hooters. You may not want to call it depression, nor will you want to talk to your GP about it as most experts suggest, but you should definitely avoid some of the other options. Bottling up your depression or seeking comfort in the booze are easy options that fail to address the underlying problem. Instead:

- Discuss your feelings with her. Take advantage of any offers from relatives or friends to babysit and get back out to one of your favourite haunts. Use the change of scenery to broach subjects that the claustrophobic four walls back home won't allow.

- Join the clubs. Online parenting communities offer new dads a chance to air their fears and concerns in an anonymous forum. If you've still got any numbers from the fellow dads at the antenatal group give them a call and meet up. They may not be going through exactly the same thing, but a trouble shared etc.

- Bargain with the boss. If the struggle to balance your new life and work patterns is contributing to the conflict at home or your feelings of despair, then talk to your HR people about the possibility of home-working or doing flexitime for a while.

Did you know?

Lost Sleep

A new baby typically results in 400–750 hours' lost sleep for parents in the first year.

Expectancy Explained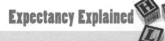

What's Worrying Her . . . Feeling Like a Failure

For a working woman, the first child especially can come as a big shock to the system. According to Jo Lyon problems occur because at work she knew what she needed to achieve and got positive feedback for it. But now she's at the whim of a tiny person who does exactly as they like – sleeping, eating and doing everything on their terms.

Often a new mother does not know how to value herself. She may feel exhausted, emotional and is probably comparing herself with others with different babies. How does she know she is successful? How satisfied does she feel at the end of a day changing nappies, worrying about how well the baby has fed? Employment specialists like Lyon point out that while expert books say you should do x, y and z, the baby is not always playing ball. As a result she can question her ability and think she's a failure.

She may suffer a dip in self-confidence when it comes to returning to work and, more crucially, simply find that the job no longer holds the appeal it once had before your baby was born. Be prepared for her to change any plans you may have had before the birth. In many cases the thought of suddenly leaving their precious baby with someone else can be strong enough for them to want to reconsider their career.

Only you know how these decisions will affect your lifestyle as a family. You may well want your partner to give up work and be a full-time mum, even if it means making some major financial sacrifices.

On the other hand you and she may want life to continue as much as possible as it did before. It's not vital that you make any decisions in these early weeks. Lyon suggests that for now you be supportive and listen. Try stepping into her shoes and seeing it from her point of view too, but most of all, as with so many aspects of pregnancy, birth and beyond, encouragement and letting her make her own decisions is the best way forward.

Did you know?

Appy Nappy Days

For fathers with a fondness for phone apps a few useful ones to install according to those surveyed on the Dad Network Facebook page include The BabyCenter and the WonderWeeks apps, which update on development milestones – other dads listed YouTube for handy tips and Netflix for an 'escape'.

WILL THEY BE OK WHEN I RETURN TO WORK?

You may be counting down the days to the end of your paternity leave – scratching a convict's calendar on the wall. Alternatively, you might have just got used to helping out with your new little son or daughter when the time comes for you to go back to work.

The transition will be a challenge. If your partner has had a caesarean and is still struggling with moving or doing certain tasks – or if she's suffering with PND or simply anxious about being left alone with the baby – then you're going to have to make a concerted effort at getting the juggling act of work and home life right.

You may have a backlog of work mounting up from your time off and demands for it to be met. As a result you could go from being on hand at home as an invaluable help for her – to being back at the office on Monday and working late. The pressure to keep on top of things, bring in enough money for all your baby's material needs and deal with the drop in income your partner will have once her maternity allowance shrinks will be tough.

Things won't be made easier if home life isn't great: if your partner's having trouble dealing with life after the birth, if your baby isn't sleeping well at night. These first few months are the hardest for all new parents. Jo Lyon points out that, for the working man, there's the struggle of the emotional pull to home, the exhaustion due to lack of sleep and the support needed by his partner. For some there's even the jealousy/fantasy that their partner is having a lovely time having coffee and playing with the baby all day long.

Lyon suggests that even before you have the baby, think through what you do at the moment at work and at play and decide which of those are really important to you. Which form part of your identity? Must they continue at the same level in the short term? Recognising that there is a life change but also a short-term change in terms of sleep and adjustment to a new way of life is key, insists Lyon. Here's how to strike the right balance and ensure the pair of you do manage to have a conversation that isn't always about the baby:

- **Plan in advance.** Prepare for the change and discuss the impact with your partner – be open with friends and colleagues about what you think will happen once the baby is born.

- **Get out once a week.** Make sure you still do some activities for you – if you give everything up you may end up feeling resentful.

- **Keep communication clear.** Lyon believes this is especially crucial when juggling work and home life. Understanding where your boss stands on the issue of flexitime, say, will play a critical role in how you influence them and the reaction you will get to taking time off work in an alternative way.

- **Study your work patterns.** Think about one or two times a week that you could do something differently – if you have to work late four days make sure you are back in time for bath/bedtime on the fifth.

- **Be positive.** Believe in what you are doing – don't make excuses and apologise for wanting to be a dad as well as a professional.

- **Get enough sleep.** Negotiate with your partner that you get some undisturbed nights' sleep so you can cope at work. In return you could do the same for her at weekends. If you have a spare room or nursery the baby isn't in yet you may need to use it some of the week. Don't be too surprised if this becomes a major bone of contention though . . .

Can I work flexitime?

Despite changes in the law permitting parents of children up to six years old to request flexible working hours (bosses must provide a strong argument against letting you take it) there is still a stigma against flexitime or 'working from home' within some workplaces. That stigma exists among new dads too, many of whom fear they may be seen as 'part-timers' by colleagues or fear they may jeopardise their place on the career ladder. If you are going to request alternative work patterns, it is important to think through the business case for this – what will make it an attractive proposition?

- How will you ensure it is going to work?
- How will it impact others? Your manager? The people you manage?
- If you have clients will it have an impact on them?
- How can you overcome this?

Try to have preliminary discussions with others in your team to see how they think it will work and what they think the barriers to success will be. Lyon suggests you sound out your manager about any ideas you have before making it more formal. Find out, in principle, maybe during the 'head-wetting' drinks, what are their thoughts and reactions to you changing your work pattern. What do they think would work?

Be clear about what you can achieve and don't expect too much of yourself. Think about little things you can do to find time in the week. One of Lyon's clients knew that their job required them to work until midnight every day so there was no way they would see their child in the evening – but he managed to negotiate with his boss to come in at 10 a.m. so he could spend some time in the week with his partner and newborn baby.

Should I take over childcare?

It's possible during the pregnancy that you've discussed changing the way you work to accommodate your new family life – but now you've spent a little time at home with your baby those feelings may have changed. The idea of being a 'full-time father' may strike you as being totally nuts. Alternatively, if you're enjoying your role during paternity leave and at weekends it may be something you want to investigate some more.

According to the Office for National Statistics (August 2015) the number of stay-at-home fathers in the UK is 246,000 – rising by around 4,000 a month. In contrast the figure for stay-at-home mums is down to just over two million – a reduction from 2.8 million 20 years ago.

The key reasons why most new dads become stay-at-home ones are financial. If your partner earns significantly more than you do, you might find the childcare costs when she returns to work swallow up most of your own earnings. Remember, in many parts of the UK children don't start full-time school until they're about five years old. Until then someone's got to be holding the baby. Nannies, mannies (male nannies), au pairs, childminders and crèches very rarely come for free. On the other hand, even if you or your partner feel you're 'working for nothing' during the pre-school years, it does have the advantage of keeping your job open for you rather than you having to find another job once your kid starts school.

Many men who become stay-at-home dads report having a rewarding experience – more than any job could ever give them.

The opportunity to watch your child grow, shape their personality, be involved in their life and in some cases become their home tutor too is something more and more new fathers are embracing these days.

Others can't hack it. Some give it a trial run during a week's holiday and hate it. Some have to do it and struggle to cope, bemoaning everything from the lack of disposable income or 'social interaction' to the 'sense of purpose' their job had given them.

If you're a dad who's not totally daunted by the thought of it and believe being a full-time father is something that could work for you both, then there are a number of other factors to discuss before you take the plunge:

Change in status:

Job satisfaction, company gossip, perks, company golf outings and 'seminars' that leave the bar dry – all the things that aren't part of the pay packet. Swapping the commute for nappy changes will mean an end to many of the things you possibly don't realise your job brings you. Are you ready to introduce yourself as 'full-time father' when asked what you do for a living?

The anxiety:

While the day-to-day job stress may have gone, kids come with their worries. Accidents, illness, teething and sleepless nights compound your worries in your new role. Some men find issues like maintaining a pension or fear that their partner may lose her job reasons enough not to quit their job for the home life.

Isolation:

As any new mum will confirm, you can often go a whole day in those early months with no conversation or social life aside from dealing with the needs of your child. While your baby may be at least a year old before you decide to take over the role of primary carer, rainy days indoors won't always be a bundle of laughs when it's the fifth one in a row.

Work from home:

It's not as easy as it sounds when you've got a baby to attend to. Right now your baby demands almost constant attention to the point where, some days, you may come home from work and your partner's barely had a chance to take a pee let alone do anything else. In the future you may be able to do some 'tele-working' but don't expect to be able to switch from a nine-to-five to a full-time dad's life and still be able to meet deadlines or work demands.

NEW DADS' EXPERIENCES

Stay-at-Home Dads

Things you should know if you're going to do the full-time-dad thing when they're still babies is that you cannot, ever, just grab your keys and leave the house with your baby in tow. You need a list of stuff to take before you take a shopping list too. Also, you won't get the shopping right for months – you'll buy stuff past its sell-by date etc. – which will lead to rows with your partner. And it's not a cruise. You don't get to put your feet up all day, even when they're little babies, you're feeding and cleaning – yourself, the baby and the house. Even so, some of my best conversations with my baby occurred when I was sat on the toilet and he was in his day rocker because you can't let them out of your sight.

'I began looking after Amy at six months over the weekends when my wife was on a course. It was useful because I was then unemployed for a year during which time I took over at home. You can go stir crazy. I put on weight and drank a bit too often once my wife was home but the actual time spent with Amy has been wonderful. You can feel a bit odd being the only man at a park or playgroup though there's more and more dads doing it. I wouldn't have missed it for the world.'   Jon C

'I became a full-time, stay-at-home dad in a small first-floor flat with no garden. I thought it would be great. I'd give classes in the more beautiful aspects of the beautiful game (football), give lessons in aircraft recognition and teach the finer points of northern industrial heritage over fish-finger butties at teatime. But I struggled from the off. Sleep is everything, and if you're not recharging the batteries then you can't function normally as a human being. According to one of my cleverer friends, the average human psyche will grind down to its basic constituents after just three nights of broken sleep. In four years, we've had just nine nights of unbroken sleep, one of which was last night. We should have put up the bunting.'   Lee G

'I never thought I'd do this but once we weighed up the options – like my wife earns twice what I do and loves her job, whereas I hated my accounts job – then we took the plunge once my wife's maternity leave ended. At first I was anxious, made a few mistakes and needed to call her at work to ask dumb questions. But now our boy is 20 months old and we're best mates. We do housework, we play, we go to swimming class and when he naps I do a bit of bookwork for some friends. It's not easy, it's not for everyone, but I think I'm pretty lucky.'   Greg H

Did you know?

Not Feeling the Love

Research by US psychiatrists suggests that around 40 per cent of new parents experience feelings of indifference towards their new baby at some point.

WHAT'S THE FORM FOR 'WETTING THE BABY'S HEAD'?

Along with weddings, funerals and major sporting successes, the birth of a child is firmly established as a reason for many a British male to 'get on it'. There's no form as such with this. If you've struck up a bit of a bond with some of the other fathers on the antenatal course you attended then it could be a good chance to share experiences – though in the main it's usually a pub or garden-barbecue gathering of like-minded mates. One very valuable lesson that every new dad soon learns via the head-wetting, though, is that babies and hangovers never mix.

CAN WE HAVE SEX AGAIN NOW?

Wistfully remembering those seemingly 'shag-fest' days you and your partner enjoyed before she got pregnant? Even if you weren't going at it like rabbits in a bid to conceive you were probably having a lot more sex 10 months ago than you are now.

In one survey as many as one in seven new mums claimed they went at least a year without having sex – during and after the pregnancy. Your partner will need to physically heal before she can enjoy sex again. The pair of you may need to psychologically mend a little too – witnessing a birth can scar a man (albeit temporarily) in ways that can put him off sex.

You'll need to take things a little easy at first, especially if she's breastfeeding. Not only will her breasts feel sore, but her vagina may be drier as a side effect of the lactation process. Couples are often advised to use a lubricating jelly during sex if this is the case. Her breasts, when stimulated, may leak some milk too – be prepared for that and the fact that many women report enjoying sex more after having their first child!

But take precautions. If you're not planning on having another child before your first one's even started walking then you should stock up on the condoms or whatever birth control methods you use. It's not impossible for a woman to conceive again shortly after having a child – in fact she can get pregnant even though she hasn't started her periods again yet. She may have problems using birth control devices and may not be able to use the pill either when she's breastfeeding – so for now use a condom or else you may be rereading sections of this book again in the very near future . . .

THE END OF THE BEGINNING

As I said at the start of this book, fatherhood is a journey that will last a lifetime. You've just taken the first few, admittedly dramatic, steps along the way. Hopefully all has gone pretty much to plan for you and you're now in what some people call the 'fourth trimester'. One thing you'll definitely notice as you wander around town with your new baby proudly strapped to your chest or sleeping like an angel in its buggy is how people say things like: 'Ooo they're lovely at that age.' It's a line that carries connotations suggesting that once they're walking and talking then it all goes downhill.

I've found the opposite to be true. As my baby has grown to be a toddler and on to now, where he's a schoolboy, the joy and happiness he has brought to the lives of me and my partner can't be measured. But that doesn't mean I don't still envy you because you've got all this ahead of you. Like all journeys it'll have its setbacks, its traumas, it can throw up some unexpected costs and a fair amount of vomit too. Right now it really is a 'lovely age' though – not only for you as parents but for your baby. Your little girl or boy is being moulded and shaped by the way you react every waking hour that you're with them. The love you show them and the time you, as a father, give them will build a bond that can last a lifetime. I hope you've found this book useful.

The role of the modern father won't stop changing either. Every new dad's experience will be different. In order to keep fathers abreast of these changes please feel free to send your suggestions, advice and own experiences to me at expectant-dad@twitter.com or my own website www.robkemp.org.uk.

NEW DADS' EXPERIENCES

The Fourth Trimester

'We got there! The first weeks are just about surviving and it doesn't matter if you have days where you don't get anything done and don't leave the house. You get through it – and it's worth every minute!'
Charley G

'Having our baby has been the most amazing thing. From the first day he was very inquisitive and attentive. I was expecting to have a baby that did nothing but eat, poo and cry. Obviously he did all that, but one look vaguely in my direction was all it took to melt the heart!'
Matthew D

'Those first couple of weeks were tough; our baby would smile in his sleep, and looked like he would have nice dreams then *nightmares. It was amazing just to have a little person at home. Also the mechanical/robot-like feeling I had for six or seven weeks of just continuous washing, dishes, cooking, cleaning – trying to support my wife as best as possible while she struggled with the feeding and emotional issues of having and feeling responsible for a new life that happens.'*   Tom L

THE LAST WORDS . . . OR . . . THE DO'S AND DON'TS OF BEING A NEW DAD ACCORDING TO NEW MUMS

One final thing! This survey of new mums, carried out during the writing of the book, allows some of the best experts and judges of your abilities as an expectant father to have their say. Hopefully it provides some sound tips – and some insight into the psyche of the ante- and postnatal female at this time. Good luck.

DO 'Change nappies. My man did and in the first two weeks I only changed four!'

DON'T 'Side with the in-laws/grandparents in general. Support your partner in every decision, especially in those awful first few weeks.'

DO 'Get hands-on. My partner pressed a hot water bottle to my back during labour for every contraction, he was a star and it really, really helped me.'

DON'T 'Think we want to spend one day of listening to crying to be followed by an evening of cleaning the house while new dad moans about everything. If said dad feels inclined to do this – beware flying carving knives . . .'

DO 'Understand that your partner only sat down two minutes before you got home and that was the first time in the entire day.'

DON'T 'When Mum gets up to breastfeed claim the next day to be tired because the baby had woken you with the initial cry! So you simply drifted back to sleep while your partner had to sit in an upright chair for 90 minutes forcing herself to stay awake and contemplating the old matchsticks in the eyes routine to avoiding dropping off and dropping the baby!'

DO 'Put up with her wanting to breastfeed the baby in the bed beside you as she can get some shut-eye while doing it. Or else bugger off to the spare room.'

DON'T 'Ever, ever say . . . "look at the state of this place".'

DO 'Offer to help with night feeds – although I never took my partner up on this as I could not express and wanted to breast-feed for a bit.'

DON'T 'Say stuff like "I was talking to the bath earlier and it said it hadn't seen you in a while"! Unlike my partner I don't get to stare longingly at myself in the mirror for 45 minutes each morning and pranny about the bathroom with no children anywhere near me! I can't even have a wee on my own!'

DO 'Be sympathetic when your partner deals with all the wakings, and has the occasional "I can't cope" weepy wobble. Take into account that while YOU'RE sleeping, she's dealing with screams. Give her a hug, take the baby and let her go off for a little while to calm down.'

DON'T 'Shout, swear, call her stupid, moan about losing sleep (after all, she does it all the time), tell her to fuck off, act like you're the only one losing sleep, and above all, do NOT say "it's all right for you, I have to go to work". This will piss her off beyond reason. She does this all the time; it will not hurt you to help for half an hour so she can calm down and carry on looking after baby while you go back to dreamland.'

DO 'Be involved from the start, particularly in the early days when neither partner has a clue what's going on! It builds confidence in handling the baby and knowing that they are doing equally well. I think that if you don't get your hands dirty from the start, dads are more inclined to stand back or feel less confident in what they are doing. Then they get left behind. It is a journey for both parents together in those early weeks.'

DON'T 'Tell your partner before she gives birth that "You wouldn't really want me there" and "I'd just be in the way" so that she is left to give birth on her own.'

DO 'Practical things like cooking, taking the baby out for a little while, cleaning, washing . . . bringing water and food while Mum is breastfeeding.'

DON'T 'Sit next to your partner while she's breastfeeding, put the TV on sports news, move the remote out of reach then go upstairs and out of earshot while we're left unable to move watching the bloody football for 40 minutes!'

DO 'Be a support – literally. When I had just given birth to our baby, I really needed a shower, but when I tried to get up to go for one, found that I was too weak as I had lost loads of blood. My husband supported me to the shower, helped me get in, and then gently washed me. I have considered him, ever since, to be the most wonderful and sexiest man on the planet.'

DON'T 'Forget that if she's had a caesarean section she won't be allowed to drive or lift anything heavier than the baby for several weeks. It's really important that you take this into account and organise things around it.'

DO 'Keep visitors away as much as possible, buy her a present, take laundry home from hospital and wash, dry and iron it and return it if necessary, tell her how great she is doing and book as much paternity leave/holiday as possible and spend time with her and the baby.'

DON'T 'Go on holiday immediately after the birth. If you do, don't be surprised when the new mum is slightly pissed off next time you phone and explain you have been too busy to meet your new son.'

DO 'If your partner, while in labour, gives you a strange look . . . arm yourself with a sick bowl before going to her. If you don't, then blaming your partner for vomiting on you will not go down well, and might just induce more vomiting!'

DON'T 'Tell people how sore your hand is where your partner dug her nails in it during labour.'

DO 'Say, "I think your tummy is getting smaller/neater/more toned all the time," after the birth, and then for ever onwards!'

DON'T 'In your excitement, email all your friends and family a picture of her just after the birth, particularly if there are any body parts or blood in the shot!'

DO 'Take loads of photos of the baby – your partner will probably be so zombified by the painkillers that she won't remember to, but she'll appreciate it later.'

DON'T 'Go out and wet the baby's head the night after said baby has been born and then come to visit partner in hospital the following morning and have the cheek to complain about your hangover to someone with a six-inch gash in their abdomen and leaky nipples. You will get no sympathy!'

DO 'Go to the appointments with her and ask all the questions that you've discussed before but your missus has forgotten to ask as her brain cells have gone on holiday.'

DON'T 'After your missus has been in labour for 30 hours and has just produced your firstborn and has gone for a shower – *under any circumstances* – eat her tea and toast. She will still be cross nearly three years later.'

DO 'Make some phone calls back home on the day YOU return to work after your paternity leave. Your partner will be petrified at being left all day with the baby – let her know you're thinking of her.'

DON'T 'Think that saying "she must be hungry" every time your baby cries constitutes a significant contribution to the support of your partner in her hours of need – remember too, having ovaries does not give you some mystical insight into parenting.'

DO 'The laundry. That means hanging up, folding and putting away as well as putting in the washing machine.'

DON'T 'Ever say, "It's your hormones, dear" – even if it is. Nor bother to ask during labour, "Does it hurt?"'

Thanks to mumsnet.com for permission to pass on these words of wisdom.

GLOSSARY

Pregnancy comes with a language of its own. It's not designed to baffle you, but in your current state of mind – exhausted, shocked and skint – it may leave you a little bewildered. Here are the key phrases you may hear over the nine months and beyond:

Alpha-fetoprotein (AFP) – Protein produced by the baby at foetus stage. A sample may be taken and tested between 15 and 18 weeks to check for birth defects among other things.

Amniocentesis – Test involving the extraction of fluid from the sac surrounding the foetus. Used to detect genetic conditions such as Down's syndrome.

Amniotic fluid – Baby swims around in this stuff as it grows. These are the 'waters' that break when labour begins to speed up the baby's journey.

Amniotic sac – Bubble containing baby and fluid that sits inside the mother's uterus.

Anaemia – Drop in the number of red blood cells the body produces, which can affect one in five mothers-to-be. The resulting iron deficiency can affect the growth of the baby, so her GP may prescribe iron supplements.

Antenatal – Any time between conception and birth.

Apgar score – Health check carried out on your baby the moment they're born testing their Appearance, Pulse, Grimace, Activity and Respiration (although the test is actually named after the person who developed it). A score is given for each between 0 and 2. Your baby may be tested more than once. Top score is a 10 (2 for each category). Most get around 6 to 8.

Braxton Hicks – False contractions (muscle movements) the mother experiences as her body prepares for the birth.

Breech birth – Instead of being head down the baby is coming out feet/bottom first. Because of possible complications the GP may suggest your partner has a caesarean section to deliver the baby.

Caesarean section – Surgical birth in which baby is removed through a cut made to the mother's stomach. Usually performed if a vaginal delivery is not possible (see Breech birth).

Cervix – Muscles at the base of her uterus through which the baby passes during labour. The 'dilation of the cervix' refers to how wide these muscles have opened and gives an indication of how close – or not – the baby is to coming out.

Chorionic villus sampling (CVS) – Test of tissue making up the placenta (feeding sac for baby in the womb). Earlier form of amniocentesis test, which can help reveal any problems with the baby.

Colic – Crying. Really bad crying, as in at least three hours a day, three days a week, for three consecutive weeks.

Colostrum – Milk produced by the mother when the child is born – packed with antibodies designed to boost the baby's immune system.

Contractions – Tightening of uterus muscle that pushes the baby towards the cervix.

Cot death – Also known as sudden infant death syndrome (SIDS). The cause of cot death is not known exactly but health professionals recommend you follow a series of good baby sleeping habits that may reduce the risk of it occurring. (See pages 220–2.)

Couvade syndrome – Otherwise known as sympathetic pregnancy, when an expectant father experiences pregnancy symptoms.

Dilation – Distance the cervix opens to allow the baby through during labour.

Doppler – Microphone used to check baby's heartbeat when inside the womb.

Doula – Independent birth 'assistant' who can provide help and support before, during and after the birth (for your partner, not you).

Down's syndrome – Birth condition that can affect mental ability and physical growth and may be identified during pregnancy through the amniocentesis test.

Ectopic pregnancy – Affects 1 per cent of pregnancies where fertilised embryo fails to reach the uterus and grows in the Fallopian tube.

Embryo – Term used to describe baby during its first eight weeks following fertilisation.

Engagement (of baby's head) – When most of the baby's head has moved down into the mother's pelvic cavity. Prepare for labour!

Entonox – 'Gas and air'. To be precise, 50 per cent oxygen, 50 per cent nitrous oxide.

Epidural anaesthesia – Painkilling drug administered during labour – if chosen – via a catheter inserted into the 'dura' cavity of the spine.

Episiotomy – Surgical incision made to enlarge the vagina during birth.

Estimated delivery date (EDD) – Date of expected delivery of baby by natural (vaginal) birth.

Expressing (milk) – Transfer of breast milk into bottle for feeding, usually done using a 'vacuum' breast pump.

External cephalic version (ECV) – Procedure whereby an obstetrician turns the baby around in the womb from the 'breech' position to the correct delivery position.

Foetal heart monitoring – Observation of the baby's heartbeat during labour.

Foetus – Stage of baby's growth from about eight weeks onwards.

Fontanelle – Soft spot in centre of baby's skull where bones have yet to fuse – nature's contribution to easing the labour pain by making the baby's head more flexible.

Forceps – Pincer-like tool used to assist with movement of baby during labour – specifically pulling the head through.

Foremilk – Thin, watery milk that forms the first 'dose' of breast milk.

Fundus – Baby's bottom when it's at the early development stage. Babies are measured from head to fundus (rump).

'Gas and air' – See Entonox.

Gestation period – Duration of baby's growth inside the womb.

Hind milk – Higher-fat milk that helps the baby gain weight and essential brain nutrients.

Home birth – Planned birth taking place at home with the assistance of midwives.

Hyperemesis gravidarum – Severe morning sickness.

Incubator – Observation cot providing heat and modified air for premature babies.

Induction – Prompting of labour by forcing uterus contractions to occur – usually through an injection of the hormone oxytocin.

Jaundice – Neonatal jaundice is a condition affecting newborns causing a yellowing of the skin as the liver develops. Usually gone by tenth day after the birth.

Labour – Process of giving birth to the baby, from the initial contractions that bring about the dilation of the cervix through to the birth and delivery of the placenta.

Lactation – Production and secretion of milk from mother's breasts.

Lanugo – Fine, downy hair that grows on foetus.

Mastitis – Soreness of breasts during feeding, sometimes caused by an infection.

Maternity leave – Time off permitted to working mothers.

Meconium – First poo of newborn baby consisting of waste (including lanugo).

Midwife – Healthcare professional providing advice and support for expectant/new mothers.

Miscarriage – Pregnancy that ends before 24 weeks.

Morning sickness – Nausea and/or vomiting that can be the first symptom of pregnancy. Can occur at any time of day or night though usually dissipates after first trimester is up (around 12 weeks).

Multiple births – Pregnancy taken to full term involving more than one foetus – twins, triplets etc.

Nappy rash – Fungal infection of baby's skin due to dampness beneath the nappy.

National Childbirth Trust (NCT) – Charity providing support and advice for expectant parents.

Neonatal unit (NNU) – Special clinic for treating newborn or premature babies with complications.

Obstetrician – Surgeon specialising in pregnancy, birth and infant-child issues.

Ovaries – Female organ producing egg that – when successfully fertilised – forms an embryo.

Ovulation – Time within menstrual cycle when a woman's ovaries are producing eggs and she is fertile.

Oxytocin – Hormone that triggers the onset of labour contractions.

Paediatrician – Doctor specialising in the care of infant children.

Paternity leave – Time off work allowed to working fathers.

Perineum – On women, the part of the body between vagina and anus.

Pethidine – Painkilling injection of synthetic morphine used during labour.

Placenta – Organ that supplies the foetus with oxygen and food during gestation (from the Latin for 'cake').

Postnatal – Period immediately after the birth (also called post-partum).

Pre-eclampsia – Hypertension or raised blood pressure condition affecting some expectant mothers caused by immune system's reaction to the placenta.

Premature (or pre-term) – Birth of baby at less than 37 weeks of pregnancy.

Prostaglandin – Lipid (fatty acid) that can induce labour. Occurs naturally in sperm.

Rhesus negative – Blood group. Expectant mothers with this are given 'anti-D' injections during pregnancy to prevent the production of antibodies that could harm the baby.

Rubella – German measles. Can cause miscarriage in expectant mothers not inoculated.

Serum screening – Test for Down's syndrome.

'Show' – A jelly-like mucus 'plug' released from the cervix when labour is about to begin.

SIDS – Sudden Infant Death Syndrome (see Cot death).

Statutory Maternity Pay (SMP) – Basic payment to working expectant mothers. First six weeks of payment at 90 per cent of her average weekly earnings.

Stretch marks – Scarring around stomach and/or legs caused by stretching of the 'dermis' layer of skin during pregnancy.

TENS – Transcutaneous Electrical Nerve Stimulation; device for applying mild electrical current to woman in labour in order to promote the release of natural painkilling hormones.

Toxoplasmosis – Parasite passed on through animal faeces; particularly dangerous to pregnant women.

Trimester – Three-month stage in pregnancy. First trimester from roughly last day of mother's menstruation (period) until 12th to 13th week of foetus growth, second trimester from then until around the 25th to 26th week and third from 26th week until birth (usually in the 38th to 41st weeks).

Ultrasound – Frequency used in ultrasonography to create an image of the baby in the womb.

Umbilical cord – Feeder tube connecting baby to its oxygen- and nutrition-supplying placenta.

Uterus – Latin term for the womb. Cavity in which the foetus develops.

Ventouse extraction – Forced delivery of a baby using a suction device (the ventouse) usually applied when the baby is in the birth canal but is not progressing quickly enough and may be distressed, or when the mother is exhausted.

Vernix caseosa – Literally translates to waxy cheese; a protective film covering the baby's skin while in the womb. Wipes off after the baby is born.

Water birth – Use of a pool of warm water in which to give birth, believed by supporters to reduce the amount of pain and trauma experienced by both mother and baby.

Zygote – Medical term for the embryo at the stage when it is little more than a group of cells.

USEFUL RESOURCES

Where possible I've included contact details or website links to organisations that you may want or need to contact during the pregnancy or the first few months of your child's life. Just as the role and the involvement of the father in pregnancy and child-rearing has changed so much over the past couple of generations, so the support groups for, the advice given to and the opinions of new fathers have evolved too. I hope that by you contributing your own experiences to me via expectantdad@ twitter.com you'll be able to pass on your own useful advice to the next generation of men in your shoes.

NEW FATHER TALKING SHOPS/SUPPORT GROUPS

Dad.info

Useful website featuring news and advice for fathers. Dad.info are responsible for the advice cards for new fathers that are distributed through maternity wards around the UK. The website (www.dad.info) features legal and work-related tips too.

Fatherhood Institute

The UK's fatherhood think-tank (www.fatherhoodinstitute.org). The institute is responsible for collating research on fatherhood-related issues, influencing public debate on fathers and their role in society as well as promoting training and support services and helping to shape government family policy.

TheDadNetwork.co.uk

Online community that spans over 100,000 parents worldwide hosting live events and exchanging advice online and via a well-established social media set-up, they're committed to starting conversations around modern-day fatherhood and how the modern dad is tackling the everyday.

Gingerbread

Parenting advice and support option info for single-parent families. www.gingerbread.org.uk/portal/page/portal/Website.

Family Lives (Formerly Parentline Plus)

24/7 support line for new parents on 0808 800 2222 (http://www.familylives.org.uk/).

ANTENATAL CLASSES

Antenatal Results and Choices

The ARC (www.arc-uk.org) is a national charity providing support and information to expectant and bereaved parents throughout and after the antenatal screening and testing process.

The National Childbirth Trust

Find your local NCT antenatal classes, including standard and specialised groups run by this independent charity (www.nctpregnancyandbabycare.com/home).

NHS antenatal or parentcraft classes

The maternity services department of your chosen hospital. www.nhs.uk.

MEDICAL RESOURCES

St John Ambulance

Run courses for new parents on emergency procedure in the event of your baby becoming ill or suffering an accident (www. st-john-ambulance.org.uk).

Cleft lip and palate

Specialist information website on treatment procedures in relation to this birth defect (www.clapa.com).

Cot death

The Lullaby Trust (Formerly FsID) Lullabytrust.org.uk.
Charity researching the causes of cot death with advice and information for new and expectant parents on reducing the risk.

Stillbirth and Neonatal Death Society (www.uk-sands.org)
Offering support and advice for parents when a baby dies during pregnancy or shortly after the birth.

Down's syndrome

Down's Syndrome Association (www.downs-syndrome.org.uk)
Promoting awareness of the issues surrounding Down's syndrome, improving knowledge of the condition and championing the rights of those with it.

Fertility and sex advice

The British Infertility Counselling Association (www.bica.net)
Resource site for counsellors and those seeking information on infertility problems.

The Family Planning Association (www.fpa.org.uk)
Contraception advice and information on options available to new parents.

The Men's Health Forum
Expert-backed advice on problems conceiving and issues such as erectile dysfunction can be sourced via their website www.malehealth.co.uk.

NHS Choices (www.nhs.uk/Conditions/Infertility)
Provides insight into what steps to take if you're having trouble conceiving.

Miscarriage (see also below for further information)

Miscarriage Association (www.miscarriageassociation.org.uk)
Information regarding what is known about the causes and treatment of miscarriage and ectopic pregnancies along with contacts for support groups and help.

Stillbirth and Neonatal Death Society (www.uk-sands.org)
Offering support and advice for parents when a baby dies during pregnancy or shortly after the birth.

Nutrition and fitness

Men's Health magazine *(www.menshealth.co.uk)*
Get into shape for fatherhood, ditch the bad health habits and learn how your diet and exercise regime can help you deal with such issues as stress and sleep deprivation.

Quit smoking
NHS free advice line and website with information on smoking cessation service and nicotine replacement products (0800 022 4332 http://smokefree.nhs.uk).

Stem-cell storage

The Human Tissue Authority is required by the Human Tissue Act to regulate the donation of bone marrow and peripheral blood stem cells (PBSC) for transplantation. Legal advice is available via their website (www.hta.gov.uk). See also the advice on stem-cell storage procedure from Virgin Health Bank (www.virginhealthbank.com).

Twins

The Multiple Births Foundation (www.multiplebirths.org.uk)
Based at Queen Charlotte's & Chelsea Hospital (tel. 020 3313 3519) and offering advice, information and support to multiple-birth families.

Twins and Multiple Births Association (TAMBA)
One-stop resource for those expecting more than one baby (www.tamba.org.uk). Set up by parents of twins, triplets and higher multiples and interested professionals, it's the only UK-wide organisation that directly helps tens of thousands of parents meet the unique challenges that multiple-birth families face.

PRACTICAL MATTERS

Baby gear

Events like The Baby Show (www.thebabyshow.co.uk) are great places for comparing the wide world of baby gear in just the one long trudge.

The National Childbirth Trust (www.nctpregnancyandbaby-care.com/home) run nearly-new sales for everything from buggies to baby feeding bottles around the UK.

Car seats can be found at Mothercare and Halfords and online at the manufacturers' websites such as Britax (www.britax.co.uk) and Maxi-Cosi (www.maxi-cosi.com). Check out the website for your car manufacturer too and see what they recommend.

Pushchairs can also be sourced via the individual brand websites – eg: Bugaboo (www.bugaboo.com) or Maclaren (www.maclarenbaby.com).

Alternatively try the high street stores such as Mothercare (www.mothercare.com) and John Lewis (www.johnlewis.com).

TENS machines can be obtained via your local health authority or from outlets such as www.tens-hire.co.uk, bodyclock.co.uk or Boots the chemist (www.bootsmaternityrentalproducts.co.uk).

To find your nearest reuseable nappy-cleaning service visit www.changeanappy.co.uk/information.htm.

Private baby scans

Firms such as www.babybond.com and www.babyscan.co.uk offer scan packages available at different stages of the pregnancy.

Working Tax Credits and benefits

The government do provide advice on working parents' rights. For advice on tax credits and child benefits plus up-to-the-minute information on Low income benefits, Sure Start Maternity Grant, Parents of disabled children, Childcare vouchers, Emergency and Parental Leave, Employment Rights and Flexible Working, Paternity, Shared Parental Leave, the Universal Credit and Employment Tribunals visit /www.work-ingfamilies.org.uk/.

DEALING WITH MISCARRIAGE

Around one in four pregnancies ends in miscarriage (often before the mother realises she is pregnant), according to data from the Miscarriage Association. Although it is common – in most cases it occurs before the 14th week of pregnancy – that does not make the impact of losing a baby any easier to deal with. According to Ruth Bender Atik, national director of the Miscarriage Association, many couples are left asking 'Why?' Because it's often impossible to say for certain why a miscarriage has occurred the trauma can be compounded by the lack of any 'reason' as such for it occurring.

Among the many causes of miscarriage are genetic issues – where the baby hasn't developed normally from the start and cannot survive the pregnancy – and hormonal problems. If the mother has irregular periods she may be more prone to miscarriage. Infection and complications surrounding how blood vessels supply the placenta can also result in the loss of a baby before the pregnancy goes to its full term.

Further research by the Miscarriage Association highlights the fact that the person most often forgotten in a family that's suffered a miscarriage is the father. Understandably the focus is on how the mother is dealing with the loss, but this means little attention is paid to how the expectant dad is coping with it. Sometimes people will assume that the father isn't as affected by the loss as his partner. A father-to-be may feel it's his place to be strong and support his partner and by doing so not reveal how the miscarriage is affecting him too. Every expectant father who has suffered when his partner has miscarried feels some form of grief – emotions range from shock and anger to guilt, failure and even relief.

If you are a victim you may find yourself questioning the 'fairness' of it all. Common reactions include:

- 'Why can some people have kids who don't seem to care for them and yet we cannot?'

- 'Why didn't the hospital do more to help us?'
- 'I should have been more supportive for her and this wouldn't have happened.'

For many men it's the sense of powerlessness that affects them heavily after a miscarriage. They have developed a strong bond with the baby, or the idea of becoming a father. They may have seen their baby on a scan and be preparing for a new life as a proud dad. Then, when their child is lost and their partner is suffering often physical as well as emotional pain, they feel unable to control the situation or practically help either their partner or themselves. You cannot take away the pain you and she may be feeling but the Miscarriage Association can provide advice on how to cope with the effects the loss is having upon you and your relationship with your partner. They have male support volunteers on hand for fathers to talk to if you need to speak to someone not directly involved but who can at least understand your grief and help you deal with your feelings.

The association also provides literature and information on how miscarriage happens and how to face the future. Both mothers and fathers who have been there report feelings that 'come and go' long after the loss. Don't be surprised if events such as friends telling you that they're expecting or even occasions such as Father's Day cause feelings of grief to resurface. Don't expect the shock or anger or tears to fade immediately. Key to overcoming the loss of your baby is communication between you and the mother. Bender Atik suggests that talking really can help you come to terms with what has happened and make sense of the situation. Don't be afraid to cry. Don't avoid talking about how you feel. Don't think that by playing down the importance of the pregnancy or the fact that it was so early on will make things any easier. Through the experiences of parents who've suffered the loss of a baby the Miscarriage Association have been able to put together a programme of support for fathers affected by it too. For more information visit www.miscarriageassociation.org.uk or call 01924 200799.

FURTHER READING

Berkmann, Marcus, *Fatherhood, The Truth* (Random House)

Duerden, Nick, *The Reluctant Father's Club* (Shortbooks)

Hallows, Richard, *Full Time Father: How To Succeed As A Stay At Home Dad* (White Ladder)

Kemp, Rob, *The New Dad's Survival Guide: What To Expect In The First Year and Beyond*

Murkoff, Eisenberg and Hathaway, *What To Expect When You're Expecting* (Simon & Schuster)

Russell, Dr Graeme and White, Tony, *First-Time Father* (Finch Publishing)

ACKNOWLEDGEMENTS

A very special thank you to everyone who contributed to what I hope is as close as you can get to a definitive guide to becoming a new father. In particular I'd like to say a massive thanks to Melvyn Dunstall, Lecturer and Practitioner in Midwifery with the Maternity Services at Frimley Park Hospital in Surrey – more importantly he's a father and great fact-checker. Also to Dominic Neary, Paul Smith, Charley Gladwin, Matthew Dawson and Tom Lewis, who progressed from anxious, expectant dads to experienced new fathers during the writing of this book. They took me back to the beginning and their time and patience has been much appreciated.

Thanks also to Marjorie Dill and Yolanda Copes-Stepney of the National Childbirth Trust and to obstetrician Dr Patrick O'Brien from University College Hospital, London. Also thanks to Ruth Bender Atik of the Miscarriage Association, to Russell Hurn, chartered counselling psychologist, and to Miriam Millar, family therapist. Thank you Jonathan Lewis of Balance Physiotherapy, Jo Lyon of Talking Talent and Sheila Merrill, Head of Home Safety at RoSPA, along with Damion Queva, Andy Tongue and Guy Bird at FQ magazine. To Tom Beardshaw at Dad.info and to the 'cast' of Dadlabs.com. Also to Richard Flack, John Lewis, Lee Gale, Matthew Barbour, Greg Howard, Jon C, Chas and Sisk for their input and insight, and to Patrick Walsh at Conville & Walsh. Thanks to Ian Allen for copy-editing the book and for being the first father after me to read it. Finally a big thank you to Miranda West at Vermilion Books for her feedback, encouragement and for taking a punt in the first place.

INDEX